The Myths of
Deinstitutionalization

Other Titles in This Series

Westview Special Studies
in Health Care and Medical Science

The Myths of Deinstitutionalization:
Policies for the Mentally Disabled
Joseph Halpern, Karen L. Sackett,
Paul R. Binner, and Cynthia B. Mohr

In the 1960s, the number of residents in mental hospitals and schools for the retarded declined dramatically, largely the result of campaigning by reformers for the elimination of unnecessary institutionalization, active rather than custodial care, and community programs as a follow-up to active treatment for the chronically disabled.

The basic objectives of the deinstitutionalization movement have been to provide treatment and supportive services for the mentally disabled in the least restrictive setting possible at the lowest possible cost.

The results of this study – based on interviews with approximately 300 individuals – indicate that these objectives often have not been met. The authors identify and examine barriers to the success of the deinstitutionalization movement, the reasons for these barriers, and their impact on clients, staffs, and the care-giving system as a whole. Recommendations are made for policy changes and initiatives that would alleviate existing problems and allow the deinstitutionalization process to proceed efficiently and effectively.

Dr. Joseph Halpern is associate division head of social systems research and evaluation at the Denver Research Institute (DRI), University of Denver. Previously, he was associate professor of psychology at the University of Denver. **Karen Sackett** is a research associate in social systems research and evaluation at DRI. **Dr. Paul Binner**, formerly a DRI staff member, is now director of research at the South County Mental Health Center, Del Ray Beach, Florida. **Cynthia Mohr**, also a former DRI staff member, is currently senior research and evaluation specialist with the Child Protection Division of the American Humane Association.

The Myths of Deinstitutionalization: Policies for the Mentally Disabled

Joseph Halpern, Karen L. Sackett,
Paul R. Binner, and Cynthia B. Mohr

Westview Press / Boulder, Colorado

Westview Special Studies in Health Care and Medical Science

This report was prepared for the Department of Health, Education, and Welfare, Office of the Assistant Secretary, Planning and Evaluation, Contract No. HEW-100-77-0107.

Copyright © 1980 by Westview Press, Inc.

Published in 1980 in the United States of America by
Westview Press, Inc.
5500 Central Avenue
Boulder, Colorado 80301
Frederick A. Praeger, Publisher

Library of Congress Cataloging in Publication Data
Main entry under title:
The myths of deinstitutionalization: Policies for the mentally disabled.
 (Westview special studies in health care)
 Includes bibliographical references.
 1. Mentally handicapped – United States. 2. Mentally handicapped – Care and treat-
ment – United States. 3. Mentally handicapped – Rehabilitation – United States. I.
Halpern, Joseph, 1940- II. Series.
HV3006.A4M97   362.2   79-27928
ISBN 0-89158-843-4

Printed and bound in the United States of America

Contents

Figures and Tables

Preface

Mental hospitals and schools for the retarded were created in the nineteenth century because it was believed that localities either could not or would not provide appropriate care for the disabled. These facilities developed into the institutions that exist today. They frequently provide little more than custodial care to residents in a structured and restrictive setting. In the 1950s, the same facilities that were constructed as an alternative to community-based care became the objects of reform.

Reformers campaigned for better community alternatives to avoid unnecessary institutionalization, active treatment programs rather than custodial care, and supportive community programs for the chronically disabled after they had received the maximum benefit from active treatment in institutions. In the 1960s, the number of mental hospital and state school residents greatly declined. In many ways the 1960s was the "decade of deinstitutionalization."

However, in spite of the enthusiasm and widespread support that the deinstitutionalization philosophy generated, the media, professional journals, and reports, such as the General Accounting Office's critique of the deinstitutionalization effort, have increasingly questioned whether the pendulum may have swung too far in the direction of community care. Most observers seem to agree that although deinstitutionalization was not a bad idea, in some respects it has been very badly executed. As a result of these criticisms, the deinstitutionalization movement stands at the crossroads and is undergoing intense reassessment.

Encouraging the maximum feasible level of self-sufficiency for all clients within the limitations imposed by the rights of individuals and the resource capacity of society has been the objective of federal, state, and local mental health and retardation efforts in recent years; however, there still exists a lack of information concerning the methods through which community-based care can best achieve this objective. The purpose of this study was to identify and examine certain barriers to achievement of the objectives of the deinstitutionalization movement, the reasons for their existence, and the impact of these problems on clients, staffs, and the care-giving system as a whole. In addition, an attempt was made to formulate recommendations for policy changes or policy initiatives that would alleviate these problems so that the deinstitutionalization process can proceed more efficiently and effectively.

Two hundred and seventy-nine individuals in seven states — California, Colorado, Florida, Illinois, Massachusetts, New York, and Washington — were interviewed in order to obtain a broad cross section of views about experiences with the deinstitutionalization process. Persons selected included central office administrators and evaluators, county/regional/area office personnel, state school and hospital staff, persons working in community-based programs, and a variety of other individuals associated with the care-giving system or otherwise involved in the deinstitutionalization process. Because of the diversity of persons contacted, no attempt was made to use a standard interview format. Discussions with respondents were largely unstructured so that they covered both common problems and a wide range of unique concerns.

Common problems identified as significant by the vast majority of persons with whom discussions were held included: (1) administrative and system issues, (2) economic or cost-related issues, (3) social issues, (4) other significant issues, and (5) the impact of each of the four problem areas on institutional staffs and clients attempting to adapt to community settings.

Problems in defining agency and staff roles and responsibilities, opposition to deinstitutionalization from within the political and care-giving system, and difficulties in accessing the generic services needed by clients were said by respondents to produce a number of negative impacts. Where responsibilities for aftercare services and multidiagnosis clients were unclear, clients were frequently shuffled between various elements of the system or fell between its cracks until a crisis occurred. Subsequently they were frequently returned to state hospitals or ended up in other restrictive settings, such as jails.

In addition, respondents stated that opposition to deinstitutionalization on the part of care-giving staff meant that some clients received an implicit message that they were not expected to survive in the community. Institutional or board and care staff also might have encouraged client dependence. Some respondents mentioned that community mental health centers neglected the needs of chronic patients, with the result that these patients often returned to institutions or somehow survived without access to treatment. Opposition to deinstitutionalization by many families and the communities that house institutions also limited clients' opportunities to live in the least restrictive settings possible.

The complexities of using generic services were also said to pose considerable problems for both clients and staffs. Services that were particularly difficult to access were: medical and dental, vocational, educational or special educational, transportation, and recreational. One respondent observed that if the client were strong enough to successfully negotiate the service system, he would be healthy enough not to need it. Other respondents described the frustration they experienced in attempting to help clients use these services.

Economic or cost-related issues were said by respondents to

be another significant source of difficulty. Since funding regulations (Medicaid, private insurance benefits, and state matching funds, for example) rather than client needs too often determine the services that are received, clients are frequently placed in residential facilities that are more restrictive than would be ideal. The result of the failure to deliver appropriate services was said by some respondents to be regression or greater client dependency.

Many clients were also said to experience frustration in the process of trying to obtain financial assistance. When financial assistance is not provided in a timely manner, clients often have to remain in institutions longer than necessary, and many regress. Those who were released often had difficulty in locating housing because of delays in receiving Supplemental Security Income. For many clients, the first month out of the institution was especially critical, and it was during this time that they had the fewest financial resources.

Clients and staff also experienced frustration when they sought community residences. Negative community attitudes toward clients, which are often expressed through zoning restrictions and fears of saturated neighborhoods, were said by respondents to have made client placement difficult in many areas. Therefore, clients often ended up living in less desirable and less resistant neighborhoods, which were commercial, decaying, and sometimes unsafe. Normalization was very difficult to achieve in such settings.

In addition, clients were often not placed in the most appropriate or least restrictive residential settings because potential board and care operators cannot obtain money for development and were unable to meet strict building and fire codes and high continuation costs. HUD funds were perceived to be so difficult to obtain that some respondents stated they were discouraged from pursuing them. The result, once again, was that clients took up residence in facilities that were available rather than in the facilities that best met their needs.

Although recent legal decisions have corrected many past

abuses of clients' constitutional rights, they have also created negative impacts for clients and staffs. Stringent standards for obtaining involuntary commitments often meant that some patients who needed long-term institutional care were released when they might have represented a danger to the community or themselves. Sometimes these persons had to be rehospitalized. Some persons stated that although they spent many hours at legal hearings, their views did not seem to be adequately considered.

Confidentiality of information requirements, while protecting clients' rights, often made it difficult for staff members to provide continuous treatment for clients released from institutions or previously served by another agency. Medication routines are sometimes interrupted or changed when records are not available so that clients sometimes regressed and had to return to institutions.

The original purposes and objectives of the deinstitutionalization movement were: (1) to provide treatment for clients in the least restrictive settings possible, (2) to provide this treatment at the lowest possible cost, and (3) to provide clients with supportive services.

The results of this study indicate that, overall, the objectives of the deinstitutionalization effort were not often met. More specifically, clients were frequently not placed in the least restrictive care environments because certain funding patterns were inconsistent with the objectives of the deinstitutionalization movement. Similarly, costs were often not reduced. When clients were forced to remain in institutions because of delays in receiving financial assistance, a lack of community residential alternatives, and community opposition to their release or were placed in settings more expensive and restrictive than necessary because they had nowhere else to go, costs of care increased. Finally, supportive services were often unavailable because of the inaccessibility of many generic services and a lack of clear responsibility for outreach and follow-up services.

Although these problems are complex and serious, many

can be at least partially solved within the current system, and they must be dealt with if the deinstitutionalization effort is to continue. It appears that other problems may be dealt with most effectively by altering the basic operation of certain elements of the current care-giving system in specific ways.

—Joseph Halpern, Karen L. Sackett,
Paul R. Binner, Cynthia B. Mohr

Acknowledgments

This publication is based on the thoughts and experiences of approximately 300 individuals in seven states visited by the project staff: California, Colorado, Florida, Illinois, Massachusetts, New York, and Washington. Almost without exception, the individuals contacted were frank, helpful, and knowledgeable about the problems faced by the deinstitutionalized client, the care-giving system, and the community.

Although the vast majority of individuals contacted provided information that could readily have been cited or quoted, we felt it necessary to safeguard the privacy of those who provided information that might be troublesome or embarrassing if it were attributed. Therefore, our findings are reported without making any specific reference to persons who were interviewed.

However, the failure to provide individual acknowledgements should not be taken as a lack of gratitude. Those who facilitated the site visits as well as those who participated in the project were gracious and cooperative. We regret that many of the views and ideas that these persons shared with us had to be summarized and homogenized for the purposes of this study.

This project was funded, at least in part, with federal funds from the Department of Health, Education, and Welfare under contract number HEW-100-77-0107. The content of this publication does not necessarily reflect the views or policies of the Department of Health, Education, and Welfare, nor does mention of trade names, commercial products, or organizations imply endorsement by the U.S. government.

−*J. H., K.L.S., P.R.B., C.B.M.*

1
Introduction

History of the Deinstitutionalization Effort

Although originally created in the nineteenth century to improve care for mentally disabled individuals for whom local governments could or would not provide, mental hospitals and schools for the retarded also eventually became the objects of reform. After years of underfunding, lack of staff, limited technology, and a general pessimism on the part of staff members that their clients might improve, these facilities began to develop into largely custodial institutions. Eventually it was recognized that to a large extent the dependence, apathy, hopelessness, and bizarre behavior commonly observed in institutions were actually fostered by the features of institutional life (Barton, 1966; Stanton and Schwartz, 1954; Wing, 1962). In other words, "institutionalization" came to be recognized as a symptom of the conditions of care in institutions for the chronically disabled (Greenblatt, 1957).

Deinstitutionalization of the mentally ill was originally introduced in response to several factors, two of which were the increasing costs and growing numbers of people suffering from mental illness. Third, the state and county mental health system, which was the primary method of dealing with mental illness until the 1960s, was inadequate. Finally, a change in attitudes and a number of events that occurred after World War II spurred a new approach to the treatment of mental illness.

The reduction in the number of resident patients in mental hospitals (which began in approximately 1955 with the in- troduction of tranquilizing drugs) is today a subject of con- siderable interest, among both the general public and govern- ment officials. This movement of patients out of mental hospitals has been commonly referred to as "deinstitu- tionalization," although to date there has been no conscious agreement on exactly what is meant by the term.

Magnitude and Cost of the Problem of Mental Illness

When officially sanctioned by the Community Mental Health Center Act of 1963, community-based or noninstitu- tional care of the mentally ill was viewed as a new approach to the problem of mental illness, which seriously affected more people as population and urbanization increased. Zusman and Bertsch (1975) noted that as the inpatient populations increased in the early part of this century, moral or individualized treatment became virtually impossible. In addition, at the same time that hospital treatment deterio- rated, the quality of life and expectations generally improved. Lower-class patients might tolerate fairly primitive condi- tions, but middle- or upper middle-class patients and their families would not readily accept such conditions.

Community-based care was a possible means of slowing the continuing rise in mental health costs and the heavy financial burden mental illness imposed on the states. As early as the middle of the twentieth century, most state governments were spending 5 to 10 percent of their budgets to sustain state and county mental hospitals and were, therefore, anxious to change the system (Demone and Schulberg, 1975).

Treatment for the Mentally Ill Prior to World War II

Prior to the mid-nineteenth century, mentally ill individ- uals were housed in various types of local facilities, such as city jails and poorhouses. These individuals were frequently abused and punished, making recovery virtually impossible. Given this situation, it is not surprising that the state mental hospital was originally seen as ushering in a true psychiatric revolution. It was hoped that the use of large, centralized institutional care facilities would mean a broader mental health funding base and relatively secure services. It was also believed that increasing the size of institutions would produce greater savings and efficiency and allow for the development of a wide range of specialized services and a large specialized staff.

In spite of these advances, mental health care from the mid-nineteenth century to the 1960s remained largely custodial in nature. As late as 1961, one report indicated that 50 percent of state mental hospital patients were not receiving active treatment (Zusman and Bertsch, 1975).

Post-World War II Precursors to Deinstitutionalization

By the end of World War II, the validity and utility of institutionalizing the mentally ill was being questioned. First, as Zusman and Bertsch (1975) stated in *The Future Role of the State Hospital,* the post-war period was accompanied by a suspicion of large institutions, from which state hospitals were not excluded. The desire to abolish large hospitals was reinforced by the optimistic attitude that mental health problems could somehow be solved (which was one tenet of the new community psychiatry specialists).

Second, institutions were attacked in a number of articles that pointed to shocking conditions that existed within state hospitals. One of the most important of these works was Albert Deutsch's *Shame of the States* (1948), which described "hundreds of naked mental patients herded into huge, barn-like, filth-infested wards, in all degrees of deterioration, untended and untreated, stripped of every vestige of human decency, many in stages of semistarvation." Later books, such as Erving Goffman's *Asylums* (1961), set forth the idea that long-term residence in institutions worsens rather than improves mental illness. Still other authors questioned the extent to which the abnormal behavior patterns of institutionalized mental patients were attributable to the hospital environment rather than to individual disturbances (Stanton and Schwartz, 1954).

Third, a World Health Organization study (1953), which emphasized the importance of community mental health care, was widely read by mental health professionals in the United States. Curious about the new approach, American psychiatrists visited community mental health programs in England, France, and Holland. They developed a commitment to patient care through short hospitalization, minimal isolation, maximal activity, and maintenance of patients in their homes whenever possible.

Fourth, and of special significance, was the advent in the mid-1950s of psychotropic or tranquilizing drugs, which were able to control the worst outward manifestations of many types of mental illness. With the outward signs of deviance under control, many previously insitutionalized individuals were at least minimally acceptable community members. Also, the willingness to tolerate deviance seemed to increase with the appearance of large numbers of hippies, yippies, and Vietnam War protesters in the 1960s.

Thus, by the early 1960s, it was clear that there were serious inadequacies in the mental health care system. The lack of effective treatment and the enormous cumulative costs of custodial care were particularly apparent. The development of new drugs, increasing societal tolerance of social deviance, and optimism that outpatient community-based mental health services could improve the quality of care and provide it at a lower cost encouraged government and the mental health profession to develop a new approach to the prevention and treatment of mental illness.

Federal Legislation Regarding
Community Mental Health Care

The first major federal commitment to community mental

health care came in 1946 when Congress passed the National Mental Health Act, which established the National Institute of Mental Health (NIMH) and authorized federal grants for the purposes of training mental health personnel, facilitating research, and developing community mental health services. Additional legislation (The Mental Health Study Act), passed in 1955, authorized an investigation of the problems of mental illness. In 1960, the Joint Commission on Mental Illness and Health, which conducted the investigation, submitted its recommendations to Congress in a publication entitled *Action for Mental Health*. Suggestions included establishment of community-based services for the mentally ill, including detection, crisis intervention, and intensive treatment. Additional recommendations focused on improving care in institutions while simultaneously reducing their size and increasing federal financial support to states and localities for mental health care.

Implementation of these recommendations seemed assured in 1963 when President Kennedy proposed a revamping of the mental health care system through the development of a wide range of community-based services functioning in the form of community mental health centers. It was hoped that the availability of these new facilities would produce a 50 percent decline in the number of institutionalized patients within ten to twenty years. Other objectives included improving the quality of care in institutions, alleviating mental health manpower shortages, and funding research on mental health. The purpose of the initiative was to work toward the prevention of mental illness and to improve the quality of care for those still requiring it (Kennedy, 1963).

Congress responded to the president by passing the Mental Retardation Facilities and Community Mental Health Centers Construction Act of 1963. This act authorized federal grants to assist states in planning and constructing comprehensive mental health centers beginning in FY 1965. The act required community mental health centers (CMHCs) to provide five services: inpatient, outpatient, emergency, partial hospitalization (for example, day care), and consultation and education programs. Additional services were optional. Federal support for CMHCs was to be phased out after several years.

The act thus heralded a change in the focus of mental health care from an essentially centralized (state-operated) to a more decentralized (locally operated) system, from more restrictive to less restrictive treatment methods, and from an emphasis on long-term treatment for mental illness to an emphasis on shorter-term, more prevention-oriented care.

Evolving Definitions of Institutionalization and Deinstitutionalization

Although the role of institutions is highlighted in these conceptualizations, it is important to emphasize the role of the community, both in the institutionalization and deinstitutionalization of patients.

Institutionalization

Originally, the word "institutionalized" referred to patients' dependence on the hospital and to the encouragement that the hospital environment gave to the development and maintenance of maladaptive behaviors above and beyond those the patient originally brought to the hospital. In brief, the hospital environment was found to have a negative effect on the health and well-being of the patient (Barton, 1966; Gruenberg, 1967; Wing, 1962). A convenient shorthand for this meaning of "institutionalization" could be "induced hospital dependency."

The patient was not induced to become dependent on the hospital immediately upon admission. Ordinarily, an extended period of primarily custodial care was necessary before the patient relinquished the struggle to leave the hospital and sank more deeply into patterns of maladaptive behavior. It was commonly observed that the longer a patient remained in the hospital, the lower the probability that the patient would eventually leave. If the patient remained for a year, the probability of release was lower than after six months; after two years of continual care, the odds of a patient eventually leaving became very slim indeed. Consequently, researchers have adopted the convention of defining "institutionalization" by the length of time a patient has been in continous inpatient care. A two-year period has commonly been used, although some now argue that one year or even six months of continuous stay is sufficient to establish a low probability of ever leaving the hospital.

This definition of "institutionalization" is based strictly on statistical probabilities and does not rely on observations of behavior. Hence, some patients who are said to be "institutionalized" will not display the required changes in behavior, whereas some who are excluded might already show such induced dependency. This definition nevertheless provides an efficient way to estimate the institutional dependence of large populations of patients. A shorthand way of expressing this meaning of "institutionalization" could be "extended residence in an institution."

The distinction between these two uses of the word "institutionalization" is important because extended residence in an institution does not have to lead to debilitating dependency. Active care and maximum encouragement of self-sufficiency can contribute much to reducing the negative effects of residing in an institution. In time, techniques could be developed for maintaining people in institutions, either hospitals or community alternatives, in a manner that avoids or minimizes negative effects. The development of these techniques might parallel those in the physical health care field to minimize the development of bedsores or muscle weakness in individuals who must remain in bed for extended periods of time. If extended institutional care is unavoidable, it should contribute as much as possible to the health, and as little as possible to the debilitation, of the patient. The statistical definition of "institutionalization," then, should decreasingly be associated with pathologically induced dependence as time goes on.

As mental health professionals have become more sensitive to the issue of institutionalization and its ill effects, they have developed a tendency to refer to any patient who enters an institution for treatment or care, for however brief a period of time, as being "institutionalized." While there certainly is danger that anyone who enters an institution may become "institutionalized," the relatively short average time of institutional treatment and the high percentage of patients who return to the community make this a very different usage of the term than either of the two previous definitions. Indeed, there may be little reason for anyone treated in a progressive care-giving system to either become dependent on an institution or to remain for extended periods of care in an institution (Bonn et al., 1975). The essential meaning of this use of the term "institutionalization" seems to be the receiving of institution-based treatment or care.

In summary, the term "institutionalization" has at least three commonly used but distinctly different meanings. Each is legitimate, but the terms should not be used interchangeably. Their defining characteristics are:

- Induced institutional dependency
- Extended care in an institution
- Receiving institution-based care

Deinstitutionalization

As Leona Bachrach pointed out, the term "deinstitutionalization" is almost always used vaguely. Sometimes it refers simply to moving patients out of state or county mental hospitals; occasionally it is used interchangeably with "community mental health," in spite of the fact that many people treated in community mental health facilities have never been, and never will be, residents in institutions (Bachrach,

1976). In addition, "deinstitutionalization" has been used to refer to the process and objective of undoing the effects of institutionalization (which has been described as learned hopelessness, helplessness, and unusual or strange behavior believed to have been fostered by a custodial rather than treatment-oriented environment).

After workers in the field became aware of the negative impacts of institutional care, they became very interested in exploring the possibility of rehabilitating patients who had been subjected to such care. Using a variety of theories and techniques, these professionals developed special treatment programs to remotivate and rehabilitate patients. A considerable number of efforts showed modest or even fairly impressive positive results. It seemed, then, that at least some of the patients who had been subjected to extended periods of custodial care could be helped to attain more adequate levels of adjustment. Perhaps the earliest meaning of the word "deinstitutionalization" referred to the rehabilitation of patients from the institution-induced dependency.

As the movement to reduce the ill effects of institutional care gained momentum, the next logical step seemed to be the removal of patients from the institutional environment. This removal was sometimes preceded by special treatment designed to reduce the level of institutional dependency, and it was sometimes accompanied by assistance or support in developing alternative living and treatment arrangements. In its purest form, "deinstitutionalization" in this sense meant removal of patients from state hospitals or schools for the retarded. As has been noted, substantial numbers of patients have been removed from hospitals with mixed results, depending on the circumstances surrounding their removal. "Deinstitutionalization" in this sense might also mean removal from one institution (a state hospital) and immediate placement in another institution (a nursing home); such a transfer might or might not improve the lot of the patient.

Another meaning of the term "deinstitutionalization" refers

primarily to the design or composition of the care-giving system. In this context, the term ordinarily refers to the provision of noninstitutional alternative forms of treatment or the design of a care-giving system that stresses noninstitutional care. Some programs have had considerable success in reducing the use of state hospital programs (Moser et al., 1975; Polak and Kirby, 1976; Sanders, 1972; Smith, 1974). Whether such programs will be successful with the full range of patients is not yet known (Bachrach, 1976). Also, it is not always clear if these programs make it possible to completely avoid institution-based care or if the avoidance of state hospital care is achieved merely by placing people in some other institution. Nevertheless, these programs certainly have promise for reducing induced institutional dependence. Investigations into the design of care-giving systems that stress the use of noninstitutional alternatives will doubtless be a major area of research activity in the foreseeable future.

In summary, at least three distinctly different usages of the term "deinstitutionalization" have evolved:

- Rehabilitation from institutional dependence
- Removal of patients from state hospitals or schools for the retarded
- Care systems providing noninstitutional alternatives

Reaction to Institutionalization

As the magnitude of the institutionalization situation became apparent, strong reactions set in. Institutions were seen by the public, government officials, and the legal system as "bad" influences on clients, some observers demanded that they be abandoned and that clients be returned to the care of their communities (Mendel, 1974; Reding, 1974). Others thought that institutions could still function as constructive links in a total chain of treatment resources (Barnett, 1975).

These observers argued for better community alternatives to avoid unnecessary institutionalization (Polak et al., 1977); active treatment programs, rather than custodial care within institutions; and supportive community programs for the chronically disabled after they had received maximum benefit from active treatment in institutions. Some client advocacy groups felt that reform moved too slowly and took legal actions that resulted in landmark decisions (*Wyatt* v. *Stickney*).

As a result, there was a massive decline in the 1960s in the number of residents in mental hospitals (Kramer, 1977) and, to a lesser extent, in institutions for the retarded (Conroy, 1977; U.S., GAO, 1977). In many ways, the 1960s was the decade of "deinstitutionalization." A recent article by Bassuk and Gerson (1978) suggested that during this period, "deinstitutionalization" became dogma to the mental health establishment.

Reaction to Deinstitutionalization

The current social, legal, and political climate makes an examination of the deinstitutionalization effort very timely and potentially beneficial in terms of mental health policy formulation and change. Recent newspaper stories and journal articles have examined the removal of persons from institutions from both sociological and psychological perspectives and have raised considerable doubts concerning the abilities of these individuals to adjust to community living, the range and quality of the services to which they have access; and the assistance they may or may not be receiving to help them stay out of hospitals permanently. Thus, some have questioned the effectiveness of removing people from institutions and the resulting impact on communities and the public. Others have either implicitly or explicitly asked whether removing people from institutions may represent a case of "two wrongs not making a right." In other words, although placing people in mental institutions may frequently have been wrong, uprooting them from environments on which they have become dependent without providing adequate follow-up services may merely compound that wrong.

The time also appears to be ripe to reexamine the deinstitutionalization effort from a political perspective. Federal and state agencies have expressed their dedication to eliminating service gaps and overlaps and many of the cumbersome bureaucratic mechanisms that produce unnecessarily high service costs. Two recent studies—an analysis of federal management of the process and results of deinstitutionalization in five states and a 1976 report of the Senate Subcommittee on Long-Term Care—have forced NIMH and the Public Health Service (PHS) to examine possible methods of enhancing operating effectiveness (U.S., GAO, 1977; U.S., House, 1976).

The legal system's recent attention to the plight of institutionalized mental patients has also contributed to current interest in deinstitutionalization. Within the last six years, there has been a growing recognition that the mentally ill have not been accorded the same legal rights as criminal defendants and juveniles. Previously, courts often committed a patient after brief hearings at which the patient was not present, and requests for *habeus corpus* were disposed of quickly. The result was that patients were often committed to mental institutions for long periods, even for entire lifetimes, without the prospect of treatment or release.

Recent court decisions have indicated that patients, in fact, do have rights, including the right to be free from cruel and unusual punishment and the right to due process. The courts have also established that people in institutions have the right to be treated or released; in other words, a person can only be deprived of liberty if he or she is to be treated. This treatment must occur in the least restrictive setting and in the least restrictive and intrusive manner possible. Other rights include the right to be treated or to refuse treatment, the right to protection from harm, the right to be paid for labor done for institutions, and the right to decent living conditions, including outdoor exercise, medical care, clothing, and public education (Flaschner, 1975).

Balanced judgments of the relative merits of community-based care and institutional care may be more possible now than in the early days of the movement, when heated debates were commonplace within the mental health professions. Trevor D. Glenn (1975) stated that social movements such as deinstitutionalization are characterized by periods of innovation, enthusiasm, criticism, and retrenchment. Mental health professionals and others involved with the movement currently seem to be caught between criticism and retrenchment. Although problems are readily apparent and competition between CMHCs and state hospitals for funds continues, virtually no one in the mental health field would advocate the abolition of community-based care. In this atmosphere, a more systematic and balanced analysis of the movement would seem to be possible.

A penetrating analysis of the processes and purposes of removing people from mental hospitals is also important now because of the need to identify major program weaknesses and to suggest remedies *prior* to making policy changes. As one study (Binner, 1977) noted:

> It is all too easy to forget that today's reforms become tomorrow's snakepits. But if a better understanding of the underlying social, political, and economic dynamics could be achieved, we might be able to institute a line of reform that has the seeds of constructive evolution embedded in it rather than a system that must respond to the same dynamic forces that have transformed wave after wave of reform into self-defeating systems. [P. 8]

A Review of the Literature

An increasing number of journal articles, newspaper stories, state and federal reports, and other studies have addressed the process of removing persons from the state hospitals and state schools to community-based care programs. Many recent publications have dealt with the controversial policies, issues, and current problems and barriers associated with the deinstitutionalization movement (Bachrach, 1976; Bruininks et al., 1978; Chodoff, 1976; Dingman, 1974; Group for the Advancement of Psychiatry, 1978; Klerman, 1977; Mendel, 1974; U.S., GAO, 1977; Zorber, 1978; Zusman and Bertsch 1975). Most journal and newspaper articles and other publications have discussed specific issues and problems relating to deinstitutionalization policies and programs. For instance, concern has been expressed over the quality of life and types of living arrangements to which clients have access in the community (Bruininks et al., 1978; Datel et al., 1978; Koenig, 1978; National Institute of Mental Health, 1976; U.S., GAO, 1977). Others have addressed the problems of community resistance and hostility toward the mentally ill, zoning restrictions, and inadequate residential and service delivery facilities (Bachrach, 1976; Bruininks et al., 1978; California Department of Health, 1974; Group for the Advancement of Psychiatry, 1978; Halpert, 1969; Rabkin, 1974).

Several publications have discussed the financial and administrative difficulties between state hospitals, state schools, and community service programs in coordinating the delivery of services such as outreach, client follow-up, case management, consultation, social activities, crisis intervention, short-term outpatient care, time-limited inpatient care, and inadequate preparation of individuals returning to the community (Group for the Advancement of Psychiatry, 1978; Kirk and Therrien, 1975; Ozarin, 1976). In addition, many publications have addressed the roles and responsibilities, conflicts, and competition for funding of state institutional and community-based facilities (Bachrach, 1976; Datel et al., 1978; Klerman, 1977; U.S., GAO, 1977), lack of training for those in charge of the chronic mentally ill and mentally retarded (Group for the Advancement of Psychiatry, 1978; Karls, 1976; President's Committee on Mental Retardation, 1976; Stein and Test, 1976), and institutional staff attitudes toward the deinstitutionalization effort (Curtis and Herskowitz, 1977; Greenblatt and Glazier, 1975; Horizon House Institute, 1975; Pattakos, 1976). Another concern has been the legal system's involvement in the rights of mentally disabled persons (*Amicus*, 1977; Scheerenberger, 1974).

Finally, many individuals have expressed concern over the illusion of deinstitutionalization. Several authors have recognized that, although the life quality of patients who have been removed from institutions has improved, many patients have merely been transferred from large state and county institutions to community mini-institutions (Aviram and Segal, 1973; Group for Advancement of Psychiatry, 1978; Klerman, 1977). When the deinstitutionalization movement began, there immediately followed the creation of large nursing homes and boarding homes in old, decaying neighborhoods where patients were, and still are, isolated emotionally and socially from the community (Chu and Trotter, 1972; U.S., GAO, 1977). In some cases, rather than being "dumped" in the back wards of institutions, the mentally disabled have been "dumped" in the back alleys of communities where facilities are inadequate and services inaccessible (Bachrach, 1976; Kirk and Therrien, 1975; Koenig, 1978; Trotter and Kuttner, 1974). Consequently, because of the policies, programs, problems, and barriers associated with deinstitutionalization, many people have begun to question the implementation, accomplishments, effectiveness, and benefits of the deinstitutionalization movement (Bachrach 1976; Group for the Advancement of Psychiatry, 1978; Klerman, 1977; Scheerenberger, 1974).

Clearly, the published material addressing controversial issues surrounding deinstitutionalization will continue to grow. However, there appear to be several gaps in the existing literature. Gerald Klerman (1977) recently stated that the gap between existing research knowledge and actual practice is immense. For example, although many journal articles and reports – particularly state and local reports – have been able to identify important issues, problems, and barriers to the deinstitutionalization effort, many of the publications lack the quantitative data needed for establishing policies, comparing programs, setting priorities, and implementing new programs and/or changing existing services (Bachrach, 1976; U.S., GAO, 1977). In addition, there are very few quantitative studies that have measured the impact of the deinstitutionalization movement on individuals' lives. Furthermore, very little research has been conducted that actually measures the changes in clients' economic and social functioning after their release from the institution (Bachrach, 1976). Few studies have gathered quantitative data on the quality of care and services, types and kinds of facilities and treatment services (particularly for chronic mentally ill and severely retarded individuals), and the need for the provision of and accessibility to various kinds of services (U.S., GAO, 1977). Finally, partly due to the lack of client follow-up research data and numerical indicators, the costs and benefits of the deinstitutionalization process are unclear. Few studies have followed the client into the community for the purpose of analyzing the cost/benefit ratios of institutional facilities versus community facilities, services, and programs (Datel and Murphy, 1976; Lamb and Goertzel, 1971; Wolpert et al., 1974).

In sum, it is evident that in order to answer many of the questions and solve some of the problems associated with deinstitutionalization, a closer look will have to be taken at the existing numerical data and the type of research that needs to be conducted. Only the collection and utilization of quantitative data will provide program planners and policy decisionmakers with the information needed for planning, evaluating, and establishing policy for the future direction of the deinstitutionalization movement.

In spite of the enthusiasm and widespread support that the

deinstitutionalization philosophy generated, the media (Trotter and Kuttner, 1974), professional journals (Becker and Schulberg, 1976), and reports have increasingly questioned whether the pendulum has swung too far in the direction of community care (Reider, 1974; Slovenko and Luby, 1974; Steinhart, 1973; U.S., GAO, 1977). This argument was apparent in articles such as Amitai Etzioni's, "Deinstitutionalization: A Public Policy Fashion" (1975), in which he observed: "It does not follow that people are better off in institutions, rather it means that if being "in the community" is to be something more than a fraudulent state cost-cutting device that results in neglect and exploitation of many of those in need, systematic efforts will have to be made to create viable, well-run, well-funded community service centers." [P. 13]

As a result of these kinds of criticisms, the deinstitutionalization movement stands at a crossroads and is undergoing intense reassessment. The forthcoming decisions will have profound implications for future developments in the care-giving system. Most observers seem to agree with Etzioni that deinstitutionalization is not a bad idea but one that in some respects may have been badly executed. Determination of the negative factors, their causes, and their remedies is of the greatest urgency.

2
Analysis of the Deinstitutionalization Effort

Goals and Objectives of the Deinstitutionalization Effort

Before a program can be carefully analyzed and evaluated, its goals and objectives must be made explicit. "Deinstitutionalization" has been defined and described in different ways by different people; however, an examination of President Kennedy's 1963 speech, the Mental Retardation Facilities and Community Mental Health Centers Construction Act, and subsequent governmental policy statements reveals that the deinstitutionalization movement has implicitly accepted five basic goals:

1. Release of inappropriately institutionalized patients from state and county mental hospitals
2. Prevention of inappropriate institutionalization
3. Prevention of readmission of previously institutionalized patients
4. Improvement of mental patient social and economic functioning, independence, and overall life quality
5. Adequate and appropriate care in communities

These objectives might be subsumed under one overriding objective: to improve the quality of life of mentally ill individuals in order to maximize their independence and self-support.

It is important to keep in mind that political factors have also motivated individuals and groups to press for the removal of patients from mental hospitals. As a 1972 study undertaken by Ralph Nader's Center for Study of Responsive Law made clear, those with a vested interest in community care have been very much aware of the upper limits of resources available for the care of the mentally ill and have therefore attempted to redirect funds from institutional to community-based care facilities (Chu and Trotter, 1972).

System Characteristics

While the specifics of state and local mental health systems and developmental disability systems may differ, care-giving systems are generally composed of varying mixtures of the following: (1) hospitals for the mentally ill and schools for the developmentally disabled; (2) partial hospitalization or day hospital programs; (3) emergency or crisis intervention programs; (4) various community residential and supportive programs; (5) outpatient services aimed at early intervention, follow-up or medication maintenance; (6) sheltered workshops and transitional employment opportunities; (7) educational and developmental programs; (8) social clubs and other community supportive activities; (9) case management, coordination, or referral activities; and (10) public information and education activities.

System Objectives

The objectives of most care-giving systems have similar objectives and include the following:

1. To provide care and treatment to the mentally ill and developmentally disabled populations;
2. To provide preventive, educational, and consultative services in order to reduce the incidence of mental

illness and developmental disability;

3. To provide supportive and follow-up services to the chronically disabled;

4. To provide quality services in an accessible, acceptable, flexible fashion under the least restrictive conditions possible;

5. To provide quality services at the lowest possible cost.

The deinstitutionalization movement stresses three of these objectives: (1) providing the least restrictive conditions possible, (2) keeping the costs as low as possible, and (3) providing supportive services for the chronically disabled.

Providing the Least Restrictive Conditions Possible

As has already been pointed out, critics of institutions recognized that many of the abnormal behavior patterns of institutionalized persons were attributable to the *institutional environment* rather than clients' individual disabilities (Greenblatt, 1957). Similarly, it was not the institutions themselves that were *necessarily* responsible for those behavior patterns that characterize the "institutionalized client," but rather it was the way in which these institutions were operated. Abolishing "institutionalization" therefore, requires the elimination of the conditions in the treatment system that foster institutional dependence rather than merely doing away with state hospitals and state schools per se.

The move to the community is primarily important not because of the change in treatment location but because of the change in living conditions implied (Aviram and Segal, 1973; Scheerenberger, 1974; Soskin, 1977). Institutionalization is not a problem of treatment location, but a problem involving the structure and dynamics of the care-giving system. One concern commonly expressed by observers of the deinstitutionalization movement is that if clients are merely moved from large institutions with dependency-inducing

structures and dynamics to small, community-based institutions with dependency-inducing structures and dynamics,
then relocation does not change the essential characteristics
of the client's living conditions and creates only the illusion of
deinstitutionalization.

Keeping the Cost as Low as Possible

Some of the original impetus for the deinstitutionalization
movement resulted from the states' desire to reduce the large
amounts of money used to provide institutional care (Bassuk
and Gerson, 1978; Klerman, 1977, U.S., GAO, 1977). The
states hoped that community care, without many of the administrative and supportive services required in an institution, would offer significant cost savings. However, these
hopes were not realistic (Arnoff, 1975; Kirk and Therrien,
1975).

Several factors made it difficult to attain the cost saving.
First, to some extent at least, institutions had some fixed costs
and costs did not always decline in direct proportion to a
decline in client population. Further, as clients were sent to
the community, a range of supportive services had to be
developed to sustain a constructive community placement.
Also, the number of admissions and readmissions to state
hospitals was rising. A larger staff was needed to cope with a
rapid population turnover. And finally, as the more capable
clients were released to the community, the residual longer-
staying population included more clients who were difficult
to manage, such as severely disorganized, violent, and severely regressed and bedridden persons. Proportionately
more staff members were needed to care for these clients
(Horizon House Institute, 1975; State of Florida, Department
of Health and Rehabilitative Services, 1978).

Two very important kinds of cost savings that have been
discussed as part of the deinstitutionalization movement are
the *shifting* of costs from one responsible body to another and
short-term rather than longer-term cost savings. Just as the

increase in insurance coverage shifted many medical costs from the individual to the insurance company, so also has the movement of clients out of institutions into nursing homes or board and care homes shifted costs from state to federal programs (Bassuk and Gerson, 1978). There has also been an attempt to involve county and other local jurisdictions in the support of services through various "matching funds" arrangements. In all these instances, the "savings" achieved primarily results from the shifting of immediate responsibility for the payment of services from one locus to another (Klerman, 1977).

In addition, the current cost picture is dominated by short-term rather than longer-term considerations of cost savings. For example, while hospitalizing someone for several months may temporarily increase costs, in the longer term, money may be saved if the person is stabilized and prevented from repeatedly entering the hospital as a "revolving door" patient. Shifting costs and attempting to cut costs (by not hospitalizing such a patient) can create the illusion of decreasing costs when there actually has been no decrease or when costs have even increased.

Providing Supportive Services

Supportive services are considered essential for helping the chronically disabled to survive in the community and to continue to reinforce adaptive behaviors (Herbert, 1977). One of the most commonly expressed criticisms of the deinstitutionalization movement in its early period was that the necessary supportive services were not available for clients in the community (Borus et al., 1975; California Department of Health, 1978; Illinois Commission on Mental Health and Developmental Disabilities, 1976). In some cases, released individuals were worse off in boarding or nursing homes and foster home care facilities where the opportunity for socialization and recreation was nonexistent. In addition, there was often strong community resistance to providing

clients with needed support services, such as community living facilities, day treatment centers, and sheltered workshops. Thus, clients often were simply released to the community and allowed to "sink or swim," with the consequent
high proportion of readmissions to institutions (Koenig, 1978;
McGuire, 1978).

Based upon the objectives of the mental health and developmental disabilities systems and the deinstitutionalization
movement, a working assumption has been arrived at: the
overriding objective of the care-giving system is to encourage
the maximum feasible level of self-sufficiency for all its
clients within the limitation imposed by the rights and
resource capacity of society (such as funding and technology). The results presented in this book provide evidence
of some of the obstacles encountered in pursuing this objective.

Substantive Impact of Deinstitutionalization

The substantive impact of the deinstitutionalization effort,
or its success in achieving its objectives, cannot be con-
clusively demonstrated. The movment has operated dif-
ferently in different states and localities, and its impact has
been examined in a relatively limited number of case studies
(Markson, 1976; Markson and Cumming, 1976; Marlowe,
1972). However, by looking at very general quantitative and
qualitative measures, we can better determine some of the
movement's strengths and weaknesses. Although they are
difficult to obtain, good, systematic qualitative indicators of
impact provide the most useful information on the problems
of the deinstitutionalization effort.

Quantitative Measures of Success

Figure 2.1 appears to indicate that the movement's underly-
ing objective of changing the *emphasis* in mental care from inpatient treatment to outpatient care has been met, despite the

FIGURE 2.1

Percent Distribution of Patient Care Episodes in Mental Health
Facilities by Modality, United States, 1955 and 1973

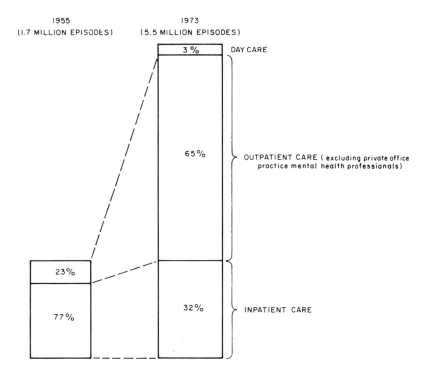

SOURCE: U.S., DHEW, Public Health Service, Alcohol, Drug Abuse and
Mental Health Administration, National Institute of Mental Health, Division
of Biometry, Survey and Reports Branch, Statistical Note 127 (February
1976).

fact that the number of episodes of inpatient care was higher
in 1973 than in 1955. Although indicators for the immediate
post-war period and for 1962 or 1963 would also be of interest, a comparison of 1955 and 1973 figures does indicate a
definite shift in the mental health care system that is consistent with the stated objectives of the deinstitutionalization
movement.

Figure 2.2 also seems to indicate that the objective of releas-
ing institutionalized patients and returning them to com-

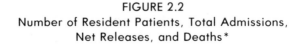

FIGURE 2.2
Number of Resident Patients, Total Admissions,
Net Releases, and Deaths*

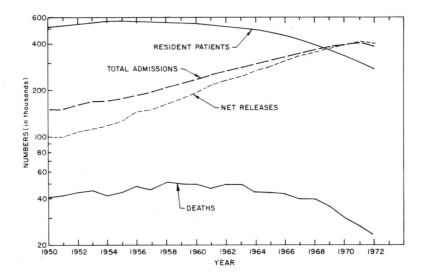

*State and County Mental Hospitals, United States 1950-1972.

SOURCE: Earl S. Pollack and Carl Taube, "Trends and Projections in State Hospital Use," in *The Future Role of the State Hospital*, edited by Jack Zusman and Elmer F. Bertsch (Lexington, Mass.: D.C. Heath and Co., 1975), p. 33.

munity living has generally been achieved. Similarly, the number of resident patients in state and county mental hospitals has been declining since 1964 (see Table 2.1). Table 2.1 also indicates that net releases and total admissions have not increased consistently at the same rate. The fact that the number of net releases increased at a greater rate than the number of admissions produced a decline in the number of resident patients. (The increasing rate of admissions is attributable both to an increase in the general population and to an increase in the number of patient care episodes.)

However, it is simply not possible to establish any direct causal relationship between the deinstitutionalization move-

Table 2.1. AVERAGE ANNUAL PERCENT CHANGE IN NUMBER
OF RESIDENT PATIENTS, ADMISSIONS, NET RELEASES, AND DEATHS*

Time Period	Number at Beginning of Period	Number at End of Period	Average Annual Percent Change
	Resident Patients		
1950-55	512,501	558,922	+ 1.81%
1955-60	558,922	535,540	- 0.84%
1960-64	535,540	490,449	- 2.10%
1964-72	490,449	275,995	- 5.47%
	Admissions		
1950-55	152,286	178,003	+ 3.38%
1955-60	178,003	234,791	+ 6.38%
1960-64	234,791	299,561	+ 6.90%
1964-72	299,561	390,000	+ 3.77%
	Net Releases		
1950-55	99,659	126,498	+ 5.39%
1955-60	126,498	192,818	+10.49%
1960-64	192,818	268,616	+ 9.83%
1964-72	268,616	401,567	+ 6.19%
	Deaths		
1950-55	41,280	44,384	+ 1.50%
1955-60	44,384	49,748	+ 2.42%
1960-64	49,748	44,824	- 2.47%
1964-72	44,824	23,282	- 6.01%

*State and County Mental Hospitals, United States, 1950-55, 1955-60,
1960-64 and 1964-72.

SOURCE: Earl S. Pollack and Carl Taube, "Trends and Projections in
State Hospital Use," in The Future Role of the State Hospital, edited
by Jack Zusman and Elmer F. Bertsch (Lexington, Mass.: D.C. Heath
and Co., 1975), p. 34.

ment and the noted changes. In the past, NIMH officials frequently argued that the CMHC program was responsible for
reducing inpatient populations in mental facilities. A careful
look at Figure 2.2 reveals that the decline in resident patients
actually began prior to 1963. It is therefore probable that the
use of psychotropic drugs, which were introduced in the
1950s, was responsible for the decline. It is also premature to
claim that a great number of patients have been successfully

deinstitutionalized when nursing homes and boarding facilities, both of which can be viewed as institutions, appear to be absorbing many discharged patients.

The evidence (Table 2.2) indicates merely that, overall, controlling for population increases, there was a rise in the number of first admissions to state and county mental hospitals until 1969 and a rapid decline from 1969 to 1972. Thus, we have a somewhat mixed picture of the success of the deinstitutionalization effort in achieving a reduction in first admissions. The increase until 1969 may be attributable to the continuing increase in the number of people seeking treatment for mental illness and/or to an increase in serious cases of mental illness. Finally, increases or decreases in admissions and releases indicate little about the quality and extent of care received by patients, whether they were treated inside or outside the hospitals.

Table 2.3 shows the percent change in the number of state mental hospital resident patients by length of stay between 1960 and 1970 and appears to indicate that long-term stays (five years or more) in hospitals declined at a rate of over 40 percent. A 1971 sample study of total admissions to state mental hospitals indicated that 75 percent of the patients were released within three months after being admitted and that 87 percent were released within six months after admission (U.S., DHEW, n.d.). Again, these figures do not reveal whether released patients were able to obtain better care in community environments than in state hospitals. If "deinstitutionalized" patients are isolated emotionally and socially in community boarding facilities and do not have access to adequate treatment facilities or to therapists, have they been successfully deinstitutionalized? If patients are released from state hospitals without adequate preparation for community living and must then be placed in nursing homes, have they been successfully deinstitutionalized? Institutionalization may occur in any location if the term is understood to refer not merely to life in a hospital but to a way of treating people that

Table 2.2. NUMBER OF FIRST ADMISSIONS
TO STATE AND COUNTY MENTAL HOSPITALS*

Age and Sex	Number of First Admissions				Rates per 100,000 Population			
	1962	1965	1969	1972	1962	1965	1969	1972
Both sexes, all ages	129,698	144,090	163,984	140,813	70.6	75.1	82.1	68.2
Under 15	3,460	4,510	6,553	7,661	6.0	7.5	11.0	13.5
15-24	19,473	25,878	37,507	35,111	76.9	88.6	114.4	95.1
25-34	22,761	25,625	26,614	27,767	105.1	118.5	111.4	103.8
35-44	23,146	25,669	30,779	24,069	96.0	106.6	134.3	107.2
45-54	19,243	21,205	24,676	19,618	91.2	96.6	106.8	83.3
55-64	13,280	14,597	18,264	12,097	82.4	86.1	100.3	63.3
65 and over	28,335	26,606	19,591	14,490	163.7	146.5	100.6	69.2
Males, all ages	72,663	82,536	98,885	95,755	81.4	88.5	102.7	96.0
Under 15	2,339	2,971	4,036	6,713	7.9	9.7	13.4	23.2
15-24	11,330	15,352	22,552	24,337	94.4	109.3	145.5	135.0
25-34	12,301	14,361	16,389	17,857	119.1	138.7	142.7	137.8
35-44	12,938	14,774	17,292	17,635	111.6	127.3	156.6	162.9
45-54	11,442	12,711	16,805	12,286	111.0	119.3	151.2	108.7
55-64	7,731	8,749	10,229	8,851	99.5	107.7	118.6	98.5
65 and over	14,582	13,618	11,582	8,076	188.8	171.7	139.6	93.1
Females, all ages	57,035	61,554	65,099	45,058	60.4	62.4	63.0	42.2
Under 15	1,121	1,539	2,517	948	3.9	5.2	8.7	3.4
15-24	8,143	10,526	14,955	10,774	61.2	69.4	86.5	57.1
25-34	10,460	11,264	10,225	9,910	92.3	100.0	82.4	71.9
35-44	10,208	10,895	13,487	6,434	81.5	87.4	113.5	55.3
45-54	7,801	8,494	7,871	7,332	72.2	75.2	65.7	59.9
55-64	5,549	5,848	8,035	3,246	66.5	66.2	83.8	32.1
65 and over	13,753	12,988	8,009	6,414	143.5	127.0	71.7	52.2

*Rates per 100,000 Population, by Age and Sex, United States, 1962, 1965, 1969, and 1972.

SOURCE: Earl S. Pollack and Carl Taube, "Trends and Projections in State Hospital Use," in The Future
Role of the State Hospital, edited by Jack Zusman and Elmer F. Bertsch (Lexington, Mass.: D.C. Heath and
Co., 1975), p. 40.

Table 2.3. NUMBER OF RESIDENT PATIENTS IN STATE MENTAL HOSPITALS
BY LENGTH OF STAY, UNITED STATES, 1960 AND 1970

Length of Stay	1960	1970	Percent Change
Total	541,625	350,276	-35.3%
Less than 1.5 years	115,548	96,333	-16.6%
1.5-4.9 years	133,038	88,415	-33.5%
4.9-9 years	96,070	44,563	-53.6%
10 years or more	196,969	120,965	-38.6%

SOURCE: Earl S. Pollack and Carl Taupe, "Trends and Projections in State Hospital Use," in The Future Role of the State Hospital, edited by Jack Zusman and Elmer F. Bertsch (Lexington, Mass.: D.C. Heath and Co., 1975), p. 53.

causes their behavior to regress and deteriorate rather than improve or remain stable.

Preventing the rehospitalization of released patients is another objective of the movement. Clearly, if patients are released only to be returned to inpatient status in hospitals, then the long-term impact of deinstitutionalization is not very great. The latest data on the readmission of previously hospitalized patients were collected by the Division of Biometry of NIMH in 1972. However, the data are extremely difficult to interpret because of definitional and policy changes that have occurred over the years. For example, what were previously defined as long-term leaves are now defined as discharges. In addition, because of the large number of patients who were released from institutions, the population at risk of readmission has increased. NIMH responded to these interpretation problems by creating a readmission index, which indicates that readmissions, as a percentage of total admission, rose from 47 percent in 1969 to 54 percent in 1972 (U.S., DHEW, 1974). However, the readmission index does not reflect the readmission rate since it does not relate the number of readmissions to an identified number of patients at risk of being readmitted. As more patients are discharged and the number at risk of being readmitted increases, the readmission index might be expected to rise. The readmission rate or the number of readmissions per 100 or 1,000 patients at risk of readmission for a given time period, on the other hand, might remain quite stable. Unfortunately, studies using readmission rates are relatively rare (McPartland and Richard, 1966). One study which was completed, in 1974, examined schizophrenics who had been removed from hospitals. It indicated that half of those patients were rehospitalized within two years of discharge (Gunderson, 1974). More studies that examine the percentage of patients returning to inpatient care status in state hospitals are needed if we are to begin to assess the impact of deinstitutionalization on total readmissions. Further analysis is also essential in order to determine whether there is a relationship between the lack of adequate community services and the possible large percentage of patients who are readmitted for inpatient care.

Generalizations about readmissions should be regarded cautiously. A recent review by Leona Bachrach of follow-up studies on released state mental patients indicated that the present body of literature on the subject lacks comparability and generalizability with respect to: (1) the interval between patient releases and follow-up; (2) the basis for release – some patients had been judged ready for release and some were released because the hospital was closing; and (3) the patient's period of residence in hospitals (Bachrach, 1976a).

Few quantitative studies have measured changes in patients' economic and social functioning and degree of independence. Such measures are essential to a systematic evaluation of the success of deinstitutionalization. For example, policymakers need to know whether patients received more and better services in communities than they received in institutions, whether released patients are able to obtain employment, whether isolation and dependence decrease upon release, whether patients' self-satisfaction increases after placement in the community, whether problem behavior decreases, whether general health improves, and so on. If we had reliable and valid measures of the levels at which patients function, studies could be done that would reveal how community-based care compares with traditional institutional care. It would also be possible to determine how the various community-based care alternatives compare with each other. However, in the absence of such measures, less systematic nonquantifiable indicators of change in the quality of life must be relied upon.

Qualitative Measures of Success

Martin Gittelman stated in a speech to the New York legislature in 1971 (Chu and Trotter, 1972):

> It is clear that we have to begin to rethink our concepts of success in treatment. Success can no longer be measured in terms of reduction of beds set aside for mental patients or in discharge rates. Untreated and poorly treated patients can be hidden in the community as well as in the back wards. . . . We must be aware that institutionalism with its debilitating effect on the mentally ill can occur outside the hospital as well as inside. The former mental patient who is relocated into dozens of hotels throughout the state, supported by the Department of Welfare, is not immune to the effects of institutionalism. [P. II-29]

Although the life quality of some individuals who have been removed from institutions has surely improved, there is clear evidence of a general failure to achieve the objective. It appears that many individuals may have left mental hospitals only to enter other institutions, such as nursing homes or inadequate boarding home facilities in poor neighborhoods, where few, if any, services are available. Many nursing and boarding home facilities are not equipped to treat the mentally ill and therefore serve a simple custodial function.

Although it is difficult to attribute the increasing number of mentally disabled individuals in nursing homes directly to the deinstitutionalization effort, this assumption needs to be tested. A 1974 survey by the National Center for Health Statistics showed the the number of mentally disabled (including retardate) nursing home residents had increased by 48 percent from 1969. It also appears that there are now more mentally ill individuals in nursing homes than in public mental hospitals (U.S., GAO, 1977).

State and county mental hospitals, which are often large and impersonal and lack adequate treatment services, have been defined as institutional; yet other facilities, not defined as institutional, often exhibit many of the same characterristics. A 1974 study by the National Center for Health Statistics indicated that 50 percent of all nursing home residents were located in facilities with 100 or more beds, and 15 percent resided in facilities with 200 or more beds (U.S., GAO, 1977).

One of the major reasons that people are often returned to mental hospitals is the lack of quality community residences and services to which people may be sent. Surveys of several state mental health departments indicated that substantial numbers of patients are inappropriately admitted to state hospitals merely because there are no adequate community treatment services. The State of Massachusetts estimated that 50 to 75 percent of its admittees were inappropriately admitted, while Maryland estimated that 25 to 50 percent of its admittees could have been treated in communities if adequate services had been available. A 1974 study of patients in mental hospitals in Texas indicated that 64.5 percent could have been released to communities if services and facilities had been available (U.S., GAO, 1977).

In addition, several problems have arisen around implementation of the original CMHC intention to serve previously hospitalized patients. A 1974 study of previously hospitalized patients in Hawaii indicated that only about 10 percent were treated in CMHCs (Kirk and Therrien, 1975). As Kirk and Therrien (1975) stated:

Although community mental health programs were established to supplant the traditional state mental hospital, both their ideology and their most common services are not directed at the needs of those who have traditionally resided in state psychiatric institutions. The ideology of community mental health has been primarily concerned with primary prevention, the importance of early diagnosis and treatment, consultation, social action, crisis intervention, short-term out-patient care, and time-limited brief inpatient care. [P. 210]

Therefore, the CMHCs have been more interested in dealing with more "normal" and "desirable" individuals who appear to be only mildly disturbed, potentially responsive to therapy, and hence, more likely to elicit counselor satisfaction. Thus, CMHCs ignore many severely ill patients.

A third problem relates to difficulties surrounding coordination and communication between state hospitals and community mental health centers. Again the patient suffers. Where releases are not coordinated, the patient may get "lost" within the complex mental health care system and fail to identify necessary services. The CMHCs are not always outreach oriented and there has been no clearly designated responsible individual or agency to maintain contact with and provide help to patients.

A related problem is that patients often have not been adequately prepared to return to community life. They have received little training in job or social skills; in many cases, training has been inadequate in helping patients overcome institutionally induced dependence. When such patients are housed in settings such as unlicensed boarding or nursing homes, they simply resume their institutional lifestyles of passivity, dependence, lack of goal orientation, and hopelessness. This reversion to institutional lifestyle may be reinforced when former patients encounter community hostility and fear in the form of isolation, arrest, or harassment by the police and when they face zoning changes or regulations that may make living in certain areas virtually impossible.

Because there is no conclusive information on the change or lack of change in patients' life quality and because the media has a tendency to publicize the most sensational case histories, we cannot draw any definitive conclusions about changes in quality of life using qualitative information. However, it is apparent from some data that much needs to be done to improve community care facilities and services.

An Evaluation of the Process of Management and Bureaucratic Coordination

Management problems plagued community mental health centers even before they began operating. Plans for the CMHCs were never coordinated because statewide planning (required by Congress as a means of fostering cooperation) did not precede the planning for specific centers. In addition, because there was a need to obligate funds within a single year, federal officials sometimes ignored plans made at the state and local levels. As Chu and Trotter (1972) pointed out, "Not to obligate all of the money and return a portion to Congress was politically unfeasible for NIMH since such an unheard-of act would have brought both the Institute and the need for community mental health centers into considerable question." Further, in this early period, there were few people trained to implement the new community mental health idea. It was not possible to evaluate and revise early pilot efforts because of the small amount of time between the authorization of funds and the implementation of the program. The results of the failure to foster cooperation and coordination are still apparent today and have been primary obstacles to the success of the community-based care movement.

The magnitude of the coordination problem is immediately apparent: 135 federal programs under eleven major agencies or departments are involved directly or indirectly in the deinstitutionalization effort. Eighty-nine of these programs are located within the Department of Health, Education, and Welfare, which is supposed to lead the effort. However, the deinstitutionalization effort has not commanded serious attention until recently. As a recent GAO report made clear, deinstitutionalization of the mentally disabled did not become a departmental or secretarial objective of HEW's operational planning system until 1976, when developing a strategy for the retarded was made a formal objective subject to monitoring by the secretary (U.S., GAO, 1977).

Evidence of the lack of coordination and attention to deinstitutionalization as a national goal is immediately apparent in the regulations for Medicare, Medicaid, and Supplemental Security Income (SSI), which in the past often created disincentives both to employment of the mentally disabled and to community living. For example, Medicaid has made it easier to obtain support in nursing facilities than in community facilities. There have also been financial incentives to the states to encourage people to accept nursing home care, since the states have been reimbursed for 50 to 78 percent of the costs. Medicare has provided very limited support for the treatment of mental illness outside institutions. Although SSI was geared to support community living, people needing temporary institutional care often lost SSI eligibility, which hindered their return to community living. In addition, in the past SSI was not available to people residing in publicly owned and operated facilities such as halfway houses and other small, frequently noninstitutional settings. SSI also could not be received unless a person was found to have a total disability expected to last at least a year.

Thus, the federal government's system provides definite incentives to continue the care of mentally ill persons in noncommunity settings. In addition, the regulations for eligibility and benefits are frequently so complex that people never learn of or receive services for which they qualify because a case management system does not exist.

Bureaucratic and coordination problems have also existed at the state level. Powerful political coalitions have frequently supported the maintenance of high expenditures for state hospitals where the number of patients has declined because of the fear of cutbacks or shutdowns. In other states, concern with expenses and the belief that dollars can be saved through community mental health have led to the closing of hospitals that are a necessary component of the mental health care system. Hospitals can meet certain needs that other institutions cannot. Some patients fail to cope in society or their condition worsens. From the viewpoint of society, a long-standing function of the mental hospital was to provide custody and asylum, both of which are still needed in some cases.

Competition for funds has often led to political conflict and lack of communication between state hospital personnel and the staffs at CMHCs. The conflict has worked against continuity of care, post-release follow-up, and tracking of released patients. Geographic dispersion has also contributed to poor communication.

Local problems have also detracted from the success of the deinstitutionalization effort. The original intent of the 1963 act was that federal "seed money" would eventually cease and that states and localities would be responsible for supporting community-based mental health care. This assumption has proven to be extremely idealistic, and congressional renewals of federal support have been essential. However, even with federal support, many cities, because of their narrow tax bases, have found it difficult to finance quality services for released mental patients, many of whom were never their residents. Some states, such as Colorado, have not been willing to help cities finance needed services, which often results in cutbacks in programs or staff. Services have then been available only to those with the ability to pay.

A brief review of purely quantitative measures of the success of the deinstitutionalization effort (such as the number of patients who have been released from state and county hospitals, the decrease in first admissions to state and county mental hospitals, and the length of patient stays in such hospitals) gives the distinct impression that the deinstitutionalization effort has been successful. However, more careful consideration of statistics and additional information on the increasing number of mentally ill individuals who occupy space in nursing homes, apparently high readmission rates, and the effect of tranquilizing drugs on releases indicates that success has not been achieved.

It is also evident, that in a substantial number of cases, the life quality of released patients has not improved. In part, lack of change is attributable to poor initial planning, a lack of leadership responsibility and guidance, lack of standards for adequate care, and the enormous problems inherent in coordinating an effort involving 135 federal programs, fifty states, and hundreds of localities.

Although deinstitutionalization has been declared an objective of federal, state, and local mental health and retardation efforts in recent years, there is still a lack of information concerning how community-based care can best achieve the goals that have been identified as the ultimate measure of its success. Our purpose is to examine certain problems of the deinstitutionalization process, the reasons for their existence, and the impact of these features of the system on clients, staff, and the care-giving system as a whole.

3
The Research Approach

The purpose of this study was to formulate recommendations for policy changes or initiatives that would alleviate problems so that the deinstitutionalization process could proceed more efficiently and effectively. The data for this analysis were collected according to the following design.

Selection of Sites

Sites were selected with the aim of providing diverse experiences with the deinstitutionalization process. Seven states were selected and visited: California, Colorado, Florida, Illinois, Massachusetts, New York, and Washington. This sample provided a wide geographical dispersion and included areas of varying population densities. Five of the states had existing community support programs; all had early and extensive involvement in the deinstitutionalization movement; and two of the states have made innovative efforts to deal with the mentally disabled. In general, the sample of states provided a good cross section of characteristics that appear important for the deinstitutionalization process.

Selection of Persons for Interviews

The selection of individuals in the seven states was geared to obtain a broad cross section of experiences with the deinstitutionalization process. Persons selected included central

Table 3.1.   DISTRIBUTION OF PEOPLE INTERVIEWED
(N=279)

Type of Personnel	Percent
Central Office	22
County/Regional/Area	18
State School/Hospital	19
Community-Based Programs	25
Others (researchers, clients, families of clients)	16
TOTAL	100%

office administrators and evaluators, county/regional/area office personnel, state school and hospital staff, persons working in community-based programs, and a variety of other individuals associated with the care-giving system or otherwise involved in the deinstitutionalization process (see Table 3.1).

Central Office Personnel

Central office personnel with whom discussions were held included administrators responsible for the overall operation of the state mental health and developmental disabilities programs, including divisional directors and deputy, associate, or assistant directors of mental health and developmental disabilities programs and their advisors and consultant groups. In addition, staff spoke with administrators of institutions; licensing, zoning, and residential facilities administrators; social services or public welfare officers; and community services and fiscal control administrators. Within departments for mental health and developmental disabilities, discussions were held with directors of special programs, including those responsible for community support programs and their staffs; institutional and residential program staffs; staff developers; researchers; budget officers; and supervisors and monitors of federal grants. Twenty-two percent of the persons with whom project staff met were central office personnel.

County/Regional/Area Personnel

Project staff also met with county/regional/area personnel. Persons with whom discussions were held included directors, assistant directors, and administrators of social services, mental health, and developmental disabilities programs at the county/regional/area levels, and persons charged with implementing involuntary commitment legislation. Also included were advocacy program administrators; planners engaged in special education; those responsible for continuity of care and interagency coordination; and persons responsible for the administration of residential facilities, including follow-up and placement coordinators. Eighteen percent of the persons with whom staff met fell into this category.

State School and State Hospital Personnel

State school and state hospital personnel represented a significant segment of the people with whom discussions were held. Superintendents and assistant superintendents, administrative aides, and program design personnel were included in discussions, as were the directors of various services and programs, such as adult services; geriatrics and children's programs; legal and forensic services; and directors of nursing, social work, and psychological services. In addition, staff met with persons who acted as liaisons with CMHCs, case managers, after-care treatment teams, and persons involved with community services generally. Discussions were also held with hospital unit or ward supervisors and their staffs, which included nurses, social workers, persons reponsible for patient follow-up after discharge, and technicians and paraprofessionals. Nineteen percent of those with whom discussions were held were employed by state institutions for the mentally ill or developmentally disabled.

Administrators in Community-Based Programs

Twenty-five percent of the persons with whom staff met were administrators or deliverers of services in community-based programs, including directors, assistant directors, and program directors of community mental health centers and clinics and their research staffs, and administrators of community centers for the developmentally disabled. Discussions were also held with clinicians and social workers and persons providing transitional care, community support, and crisis or outreach services or services designed to keep chronic patients from returning to the hospital. Project staff also met with inpatient hospital services personnel within CMHCs or their contracting organizations. Community residential facility personnel were also contacted, including administrators and staffs of board and care facilities, intermediate care facilities, halfway houses, group homes, sheltered workshops, and day care centers. Finally, staff met with administrators of specially constructed private services organizations to serve chronic patients who had "dropped out" of the existing system and advocates for deinstitutionalized persons, such as directors of associations for retarded citizens.

Others Selected for Interviews

Other persons with whom discussions were held included university researchers in both mental health and developmental disabilities, clients, and families of clients. Sixteen percent of the respondents fell into this category.

In total, 279 persons were contacted on site, either individually or in groups. In addition, respondents provided a variety of documents that amplified the material covered in the discussions.

Discussion Format

Because of the diversity of persons contacted, no attempt

was made to impose a standard interview format. Prior to on-site discussions, the research staff usually provided only a brief explanation of their identity and organizational affiliation and expressed interest in the individual's involvement with the deinstitutionalization process. In order to maximize the likelihood that individuals would share their views of the most pressing problems that they faced and their own experiences with the deinstitutionalization process, discussions were deliberately designed to be open, unstructured, and confidential.

Discussions ordinarily revolved around the discussant's current involvement with the deinstitutionalization effort. Subsequently, project staff asked about specific problems, possible solutions, and the impact of these problems on clients.

Because the discussions with each respondent were largely unstructured, they covered a wide range of unique concerns, as well as a number of common topics. For instance, many central office personnel were concerned with issues such as administrative roles and functions and funding patterns; service providers were more likely to discuss their views of problems and barriers to direct services for their clients. Thus, on the one hand, the positions that individuals held clearly dictated their areas of concern, which meant that discussions revealed a variety of attitudes and perspectives on important problems involved in the deinstitutionalization process. On the other hand, many respondents, especially those currently holding central or regional office positions, had previously been involved in the deinstitutionalization process in other capacities; for this reason, many direct-service providers and administrators were able to address the same issues.

Although discussions were held with 279 persons, not all of the interviews were documented in sufficient detail to be fully analyzed for the issues examined in the following chapters. For example, several discussions with clients and their families could not reasonably be recorded. A total of 237 interviews resulted in materials that were later subjected to detailed analysis. Views of the remaining 42 persons are reflected throughout this report.

For the purposes of our analysis, the major issues discussed with respondents are grouped into five categories: (1) *administrative and system issues* that were said by respondents to have a definite impact on the deinstitutionalization process; (2) *economic or cost-related issues* that surfaced during discussions with representative or virtually all system elements; (3) *social issues*, involving relationships between deinstitutionalized clients and the community; (4) *other significant issues*; and (5) the *impact* of all of these issues. To the extent possible, quantitative as well as descriptive indications of findings have been provided. The tables included in the following section indicate the major issues that respondents discussed, the total number of respondents discussing each issue, and the percentage of all 237 respondents who felt the issue represented a problem.

4
Results of the Study

Administrative and System Issues

A significant number of respondents who held either administrative or service delivery positions identified systemic barriers to the achievement of the objectives set forth by the deinstitutionalization movement. Three primary problem areas were identified: difficulties in defining agency and staff roles and responsibilities, opposition to deinstitutionalization from within the political and care-giving system, and difficulties experienced in attempting to use various generic services (see Table 4.1).

Agency and Staff Roles and Responsibilities

The intent of the deinstitutionalization movement was to transfer the responsibility for mentally ill and mentally retarded clients from institutions to the community. However, frequently this transfer does not occur. While responsibility previously was centrally located in the institution, it is now fragmented among a number of agencies and/or is difficult to assign to a specific element within the care-giving system. Sixty percent of all respondents (N = 237) noted that agency and staff roles and responsibilities were a problem.

While a variety of problems that will be discussed elsewhere might also be addressed here, this section will focus on only two specific areas of difficulty that respondents mentioned: (1) responsibility for the care of the multidiagnosis

Table 4.1. ADMINISTRATIVE AND SYSTEM ISSUES

	Discussed Issue	Percentage of all respondents (N=237) identifying problem
	N	%
Agency and Staff Roles and Responsibilities	144	60
Multi-Problem	80	34
Aftercare/Follow-up Services	107	44
System Opposition to Deinstitutionalization	166	68
Hospital/School Staff	85	32
Families of Clients	57	21
CMHC Staff	105	42
Host Communities	34	13
Other Agencies and Staff	52	19
Difficulties in Using Generic Services	182	74
Medical/Dental	99	38
Vocational Training/Placement	111	45
Education/Special Education	51	20
Transportation	68	28
Socialization/Recreational Activities	53	20

client; and (2) coordination of aftercare and follow-up services.

The Multidiagnosis Client. Thirty-four percent of the total number of respondents felt that multiproblem or multidiagnosis clients were particularly likely to "fall between the cracks" or to be shuffled between system elements when roles and responsibilities were not clear. Respondents identified mentally ill retarded persons, mentally retarded offenders, and mentally ill substance abusers as multidiagnosis clients who were especially likely to be negatively affected because no agency saw itself as having primary responsibility for meeting their needs. To some extent this absence of clear responsibility was due to a lack of knowledge of how to deal with these clients.

Multidiagnosis clients tend to be particularly difficult and do not easily fit into treatment programs designed for clients with clearer diagnoses. Respondents observed that clients who were both mentally ill and mentally retarded experienced particular problems in using mental health services. Sometimes they found themselves inappropriately placed in insight-oriented group therapy with nonretarded clients. More often they found the mental health system reluctant to exercise adequate responsibility for their mental health problems; and the developmental disability system regarded their mental health needs as outside its domain.

Finally, there appeared to be no particular incentives to care-giving systems for dealing with these clients, and responsibility questions often revolved around who should bear the cost of serving them.

In general, then, the multidiagnosis client was considered difficult to place in standard programs for either the mentally ill or the mentally retarded and suffered considerable rejection within the care-giving system. Ways of training staffs and funding programs – such as therapy, vocational programs, and social and recreational activities – to deal with the special needs of multiple diagnosis groups should be developed.

Aftercare and Follow-Up Services. The delivery of aftercare and follow-up services was viewed as a problem by 44 percent of all respondents. As would be expected, clients were most likely to be "lost" when they left the hospital or state school and entered the community service system. For example, mental patients may have experienced difficulty in getting medications after they left the hospital. Staff members became frustrated when they felt that they were fulfilling roles that more appropriately belonged to the mental health center or, conversely, to the state hospital. Other questions arose about which agencies and staff should be involved in discharge planning and at what point they should have become involved. Many outreach and case management programs that are oriented to follow-up services were funded with "soft" money and were staffed temporarily by, for example, CETA (Comprehensive Employment and Training Act) positions. Thus, clients may have experienced serial relationships with the staff, which made it more difficult for them to remain in the community.

Suggestions for Improving the System. The most common suggestion for helping clients to maximize their benefits from the system was to provide a buffer in the form of a case manager. The case manager might control the resources needed to provide services, assist the client through a particular administrative procedure, or help to locate needed services. Most respondents agreed that it was not adequate, in most cases, merely to refer the client to another agency or staff member, to send a letter to the client or another agency, or to suggest a general course of action for the client.

Higher level administrators often suggested other solutions to system problems, including greater administrative coordination through umbrella agencies, regional responsibility for all services, or other administrative devices. However, many direct-service providers rejected such administrative solutions since they would merely produce more administrative structures that would hinder provision of client services.

It seems clear that aftercare and follow-up services have often not been the responsibility of any particular agency or individuals so that clients experienced difficulty in the process of moving from the institution to the community and then remaining in the community. Responsibility for aftercare services should be more clearly defined; case-management–oriented programs should be given priority status; and longer-term funding mechanisms should be initiated.

System Opposition to Deinstitutionalization

Sixty-eight percent of all respondents stated that there was resistance to or skepticism of the deinstitutionalization process. Some persons expressed a limited endorsement of the deinstitutionalization effort and their frustration with its realities as compared to the goals it was originally designed to achieve. Most respondents were concerned about the way in which deinstitutionalization had been implemented: moving clients out of institutions to settings that were inappropriate for their needs and/or that were more restrictive than necessary. Respondents stated that the problems of deinstitutionalization were attributable both to the lack of funds for follow-up of clients in the community and to the initial haphazard removal of clients from institutions. Much of the early deinstitutionalization effort was described as having been undertaken with little planning and under considerable administrative and political pressure.

The following categories of persons were identified as having resisted the process of deinstitutionalization: (1) hospital or school staffs, (2) families of clients, (3) CMHC staffs, (4) host communities, and (5) other agencies and staffs.

Hospital or School Staffs. The staffs of institutions were mentioned by 32 percent of all respondents as a significant force opposed to deinstitutionalization. One obvious reason for institutional resistance to deinstitutionalization was the threat of job loss. However, institutional respondents were not only concerned about their jobs but were also unhappy at being told that their efforts were no longer needed. Institutional staff members also stressed their concern that clients were not being well served by the process of deinstitutionalization. For example, in one state an extensive media campaign by employees of institutions charged that patients were being "dumped" as a matter of political expediency.

Some members of hospital staffs also expressed their concern over the adequacy and availability of hospital services. Many of them were frustrated that, because of legalities, some patients had been only partially treated when they were released into the community. In addition, the number of hospital personnel was reduced, even though many cases were more difficult. Although institutional respondents felt that they were expected to provide quality care, many asserted that a return to custodial care would inevitably result from staff cutbacks.

It is reasonable to conclude that institutional staff members felt threatened by the deinstitutionalization movement. Motivated by personal economics and concern for patients' welfare, institutional employees were resistant to the process of relocating patients in the community. The impact of job loss could be reduced by providing funds and work incentives for employee retraining, relocation, and the transfer of benefits.

Families of Clients. Twenty-one percent of all respondents stated that the families of clients opposed deinstitutionalization efforts. While respondents occasionally mentioned that opposition existed among the families of the mentally ill, positive responses were obtained primarily from persons who discussed the families of the mentally retarded.

To many parents of the retarded, the institution represented a secure haven. Particularly as parents grow older and realize that they will not be able to protect the interests of their children indefinitely, they expressed concern about placement in the community. Respondents were concerned that community facilities might close or that they might vary and change in quality of care provided.

A less common theme was the guilt that some parents felt about having their children cared for in foster homes or other residential facilities in the community. Parents, who had originally been urged to give up their children and place them in institutions because institutions were the only places in which adequate care could be given, were now told that an ordinary home could provide adequate care. Some persons felt there was a great need to educate obstetricians and pediatricians so that they could give more adequate counseling to parents of developmentally disabled children in order that placement decisions could be made with a longer-term perspective.

Thus, largely because of a lack of confidence in the stability, adequacy, and quality of long-term community placements, families of the mentally disabled sometimes opposed deinstitutionalization. Quality monitoring of community placements is essential if the families of deinstitutionalized clients are to accept that deinstitutionalization is in their relatives' best interests, and educational efforts are needed to improve the early counseling for parents of mentally disabled children so that placement decisions can be made with a longer-term perspective.

Community Mental Health Center Staffs. Forty-two percent of all respondents felt that the CMHC staffs did not completely support deinstitutionalization. Some CMHC staff members expressed concerns that were similar to those expressed by institutional personnel—that the community care received by clients might not be adequate. Some staff members also wished that institutions would keep clients longer and prepare them more adequately for placement in the community.

Some non-CMHC respondents stated that CMHC staffs resisted deinstitutionalization efforts because they did not know how to deal with chronic patients, did not gear their programs to the needs of chronic patients, and did not find chronic patients a rewarding group with which to work. Some respondents expressed dismay that chronic patients who did not keep appointments were often dropped with little or no attempt at outreach. Delays in providing appointments for newly released patients were also mentioned as an example of the insensitivity of CMHC staffs.

One respondent's comment sums up the perceptions of outsiders to CMHC resistance to serving clients:

> Expecting the chronically mentally ill patient to use the current mental health system is like expecting a paraplegic to use stairs. Stairs are there and are useful for people who can use them but a paraplegic can't negotiate stairs. The chronic long-term mentally ill person can't use the current mental health system because it's oriented towards people who have motivation, who have the capacity to develop insights, to change behaviors, to accommodate through socially acceptable behaviors. What we find is that these individuals are really much worse off than they were in institutions.

While few respondents argued that deinstitutionalized clients were worse off in the community than they are in institutions, they did tend to agree that the current CMHC system was not optimally responsive to the needs of the chronic patient and that clients did suffer from this nonresponsiveness.

In general, many members of the CMHC staffs are not trained or motivated to serve the chronically disabled client. Although CMHC programs were often seen as not actively supporting chronic or severely disabled clients, significant exceptions were found. Support for training of CMHC staffs to better deal with the chronic patient should be provided, and the incentive structure of CMHCs should be carefully reviewed and, if found to be inconsistent with the goals of the deinstitutionalization movement, it should be restructured.

"Restructuring" could mean broadening the range of incentives rather than merely reversing the incentive pattern.

Host Communities. Thirteen percent of all respondents mentioned that communities in which institutions scheduled for closure or cutback were based resisted the deinstitutionalization process. While the protests from the host communities sometimes focused on the welfare of clients, resistance to the massive economic impact of deinstitutionalization was at least equally important, particularly in rural communities that developed essentially to support institutions. Well-organized protests from host communities were able to affect legislative actions significantly.

Respondents also discussed the heavy local impact that placement of deinstitutionalized persons with no ties or support could have on host communities. The financial burden of supporting these persons and the frequent oversaturation of host community neighborhoods also contributed to resistance.

In sum, economic reasons and fears of negative social impacts contributed to host communities' opposition to the process of deinstitutionalization. Planners must recognize host communities' economic dependency on institutions and should consider deinstitutionalization's possible economic and social impact on the communities.

Other Agencies and Staffs. Nineteen percent of all the persons with whom discussions were held mentioned specific agencies or staffs that presented barriers to achievement of the movement's goals. More specifically, a number of respondents believed that state legislatures effectively opposed deinstitutionalization by failing to fund necessary community programs and by their continued support of the physical maintenance of institutional facilities.

Respondents also criticized the federal government for its failure to clearly plan and set goals for the deinstitutionalization movement; they stated that federal funding patterns dictated which services clients received. People in a number of states expressed their frustration with trying to meet what they perceived as rigid federal guidelines without necessary federal funds. (More detailed discussion of the perceived federal barriers to deinstitutionalization will be discussed with cost-related issues.) But, in general, federal staffs and agencies were said to have created obstacles to the realization of deinstitutionalization goals. Specific federal incentives for deinstitutionalization should be provided to states so that legislatures and central office personnel are rewarded for further developing community programs rather than supporting the maintenance of institutional-type settings.

Difficulties in Using Generic Services

At least since the onset of the services integration movement, fragmentation of the human services system has been viewed as a major obstacle for clients with multiple problems and multiple service needs. Both mentally ill and mentally retarded clients who have been deinstitutionalized have multiple problems and needs, many of which must be dealt with through the generic service system. Most of the persons with whom discussions were held agreed that services fragmentation or the absence of interagency cooperation, communication, and coordination negatively influenced the operation of the deinstitutionalization process.

Respondents indicated that the service system was integrated around the specific services that fell within the turf of generic agencies or specialized professions rather than around the needs of clients. They did not believe that the costs of successfully accessing these separate services had been calculated or taken into consideration when community care systems were established.

A sizable majority (74 percent) of all respondents agreed that they had personally experienced difficulties in dealing with various elements of the generic services system, and many could provide examples of specific problems that clients had encountered. Reasons given for difficulties included the categorical nature of the service system (with the

existence of different eligibility criteria in different systems),
turf and resource allocation problems, unwillingness to accept service responsibility for or a lack of awareness of the
special needs of clients, and the complex nature of the system
in conjunction with the inability of deinstitutionalized clients
to access the system.

Several generic services were mentioned specifically as
particularly difficult to use: (1) medical and/or dental, (2)
vocational placement and/or training, (3) education or special education, (4) transportation, and (5) socialization/recrea-
tional activities.

Medical and/or Dental Services. Thirty-eight percent of all
respondents stated that they had experienced problems in obtaining medical and dental services. A few respondents felt
that doctors and dentists were uncomfortable treating mentally retarded clients, perhaps because they feared being sued
if they made an error in treatment or perhaps because they
were unfamiliar with the combinations of drugs that were
often prescribed for these clients.

Continuing education efforts, targeted at medical and dental professionals likely to deal with deinstitutionalized clients, should be included as part of the community support
overhead costs for these clients. University Affiliated Facilities (UAF) could play a key role in developing and facilitating
these educational efforts through their multidisciplinary
training programs.

Vocational Placement and/or Training. Forty-five percent of
all respondents mentioned that the vocational rehabilitation
(VR) system was not geared to the needs of deinstitutionalized clients. Many of the persons with whom discussions
were held felt that VR staffs were unfamiliar with the special
needs of the mentally disabled, and the remarks of some respondents seemed to indicate that the VR system's emphasis
on serving the handicapped was directed toward the physically rather then the mentally handicapped.

While some respondents were critical of the VR system

because of its failure to place clients in "real" (competitive) jobs, the majority felt that clients needed some sort of prevocational or noncompetitive employment opportunities. A large number of respondents observed that space in sheltered workshops was scarce and that workshop positions were not always geared to client needs. Some respondents reported that both mentally ill and mentally retarded clients were bored and felt that their abilities were not recognized in many sheltered workshop settings. A number of persons also stated that mixing mentally ill and mentally retarded clients created problems. Neither group could comfortably identify with the specific handicap of the other, and a number of respondents stated that clients felt humiliated when they were mixed in workshop settings.

One important cause of dissatisfaction with vocational rehabilitation services was management's evaluation of counselors based on the number of clients "successfully rehabilitated." This mandate was seen as a disincentive to serving the deinstitutionalized client who could not be easily placed. Respondents also believed that, because of large caseloads, counselors found it difficult to become familiar with the special needs of their mentally disabled clients.

Respondents believed that since deinstitutionalized clients were being inadequately served by the vocational rehabilitation system, a larger number and range of prevocational services should be made available. The management evaluation system for counselors should be reviewed and restructured if it is systematically discouraging the delivery of services to the mentally disabled.

Education or Special Education. Although only 20 percent of all respondents discussed educational services, a number of complaints were voiced about the difficulty of dealing with local school districts and special education personnel. Major difficulties revolved around the cost of providing needed services to clients, particularly since some school districts only provided services until the mentally retarded reached an age above the maximum to qualify for educational services, which in most states ranges from eighteen to twenty-one. This restriction was a problem for some older clients.

Both funding and program policies for educational services to the mentally disabled, particularly adults, should be reviewed for adequacy of coverage – specifically, recently enacted federal legislation. The Education for All Handicapped Children Act, for example, limits funding to those under twenty-one years of age. The act could be extended to include all persons, regardless of age.

Transportation. Transportation surfaced as a problem in discussions with 28 percent of all respondents. Many persons stated that the absence of adequate public transportation contributed to the difficulty of accessing generic services or utilizing the resources of community mental health centers. Because of their poverty status, most clients critically needed access to public transportation. In addition, public transportation called for a level of motivation and living skills that exceeded the abilities of many clients.

Providing training in living skills (such as how to use a transportation system) is crucial if deinstitutionalized clients are to function adequately. Such training should be part of any routine package of community support services. In addition, special transportation services based on the needs of clients should be provided.

Socialization/Recreational Activities. Twenty percent of all respondents indicated that socialization and recreational services were lacking or inadequate. Some attempts have been made to provide special recreational opportunities for chronic mental patients through drop-in centers and for both the chronic population and the retarded through arranged activities; but the opportunities to use community facilities without supervision varies from area to area. These opportunities were also limited by the usually low income levels of clients and their inability to finance entertainment or to transport themselves to activities. However, without this type of stimulation, clients were generally reported to regress or to become involved in antisocial activities to combat their boredom and loneliness.

Support for socialization and recreational opportunities should be encouraged and developed in the area of community-based services. Community service employees should further the development of programs that involve deinstitutionalized clients in community recreational and social activities.

Conclusion

The results of our interviews provided evidence of the complexity of the service system with which deinstitutionalized clients must deal if they are to achieve maximum self-sufficiency in a community setting. The fragmentation of essential services, the lack of clarity of staff roles in the mental health and developmental disabilities systems, and the difficulties involved in providing holistic services to clients with multiple needs all present problems when the objectives of the deinstitutionalization movement are pursued.

Thus, we recommend that the development of case management services be encouraged as part of the effort to provide community support for chronically disabled individuals. Consideration should be given to providing special funds for these services, training service providers in the case management concept, and making the monitoring of client goal achievement a more integral part of the current care-giving system.

Economic and Cost-Related Issues

Although the economics of the deinstitutionalization process is closely related to the issue of system design and operation, funding patterns will be dealt with separately since several respondents discussed financial or cost-related issues and their specific impact on the care-giving system and the

client (see Table 4.2). This section summarizes three economic issues that were discussed with respondents: (1) federal
funding patterns, (2) SSI benefits, and (3) other financial assistance programs.

Federal Funding Patterns

Seventy-five percent of all respondents stated that they encountered difficulties due to funding patterns. Although respondents were not asked to comment in detail on specific
regulations, they gave rather consistent general impressions
of how funding patterns affected client care. Most comments
centered around federal regulations, such as Medicaid, Title
XX, and SSI (SSI will be discussed separately).

Respondents frequently commented that funding and
policy decision patterns were inconsistent and inflexible. A
significant number of individuals felt that Medicaid in particular was a disincentive to deinstitutionalization and adequate aftercare in the community. One Medicaid regulation
states that if 50 percent or more of the residents of a community care facility are defined as mentally ill, then the facility may not receive Medicaid payments; this is, in fact, a dis-

Table 4.2. ECONOMIC OR COST-RELATED ISSUES

		Discussed Issue	Percentage of all respondents (N=237) identifying problem
		N	%
Funding Patterns		180	75
Delays in SSI Benefits		116	42
One month or less	1%		
More than one month but less than three months	11%		
More than three months but less than six months	18%		
Six or more months	2%		
No estimate given	68%		
Other Financial Assistance		103	43

incentive to community facilities both to accept the mentally
ill and to create programs for them. Some individuals felt that
Medicaid regulations were too rigid and inflexible. For example, Medicaid requirements for elevators, sprinkler systems,
and flashing exit signs were said to make virtually impossible
the creation of normalized environments for clients. In addition, some private community hospitals refused to take
Medicaid patients as long as they could fill their beds with
persons whose private insurers paid higher daily rates than
Medicaid. Thus, clients often returned unnecessarily to dis-
tant institutions and were cut off from their families and
other sources of social support. These restrictions were seen
as ultimately costing more and keeping individuals in more
restricted environments than may have been necessary.

Title XX funds have enabled communities to develop many
services for the mentally disabled; however, a number of individuals encountered problems in attempting to use these
funds efficiently in their states. For example, many said that
the programs and services that used Title XX funds did not
meet the service needs of the mentally disabled. In other
words, Title XX funds were too limited and tended to dictate
the services clients used. In addition, some respondents mentioned that Title XX funds simply increased the fragmentation of services. Consequently, clients were continuously
shuffled from agency to agency, and ultimately many were
unable to get the services they needed.

Many individuals involved in the deinstitutionalization effort initially felt it would be less expensive to care for the
mentally disabled in the community than in institutions.
However, recently a number of people have questioned
whether costs have, in fact, been lowered. Consequently,
many individuals discussed the problems that inadequate
and restrictive funding posed for the development of
community-based services. For example, some individuals
said that state institutions and community-based services
competed for funds to upgrade the quality of the staff and

facilities. Respondents also stated that services were often unnecessarily duplicated. They felt that some clients were over-served while others were neglected. As a result, several respondents indicated that where costs were greater and more money was needed, appropriate services were often lacking.

A recurring complaint was that funding patterns were too closely linked to a kind or range of service rather than to the needs of clients. Consequently, clients received whatever services could be funded, rather than whatever services were most appropriate. Efforts should be made to provide enough flexibility in funding regulations to allot monies to best meet client needs, while maintaining safeguards on the fiscal integrity of the funding mechanisms.

Problems with Supplemental Security Income

The first step in preparing individuals for community living involves obtaining income or financial assistance so that a place to live, medications, food, and other necessities may be afforded. The major source of income for deinstitutionalized clients is Supplemental Security Income (SSI), which is generally acquired after a time period during which individuals are supported by public welfare or assistance dispensed by states. These payments are reimbursed after SSI is obtained.

Forty-two percent of all respondents stated that they experienced delays of some sort in obtaining SSI benefits for clients. Most of the individuals discussing delays were in the field of mental health as opposed to mental retardation. One percent stated that waits were one month or less; 11 percent said that the delay lasted between one month and three months; 18 percent waited for more than three months but less than six months; and 2 percent estimated that the delays were six months or more in length. Sixty-eight percent of respondents who stated that delays occurred gave no estimate of the length of the SSI delays.

Many people evidenced considerable frustration over delays in obtaining SSI, and some stated that obtaining SSI benefits was the major problem that they faced in deinstitutionalizing clients. Respondents perceived the process of obtaining SSI as one in which the client was systematically discouraged and rejected, so that assistance could only be secured through tenacious persistence. Some clients were said to have been traumatized by this procedure.

Many respondents observed that they had little, if any, understanding of the delays in obtaining SSI or of the mechanisms by which eligibility was determined. The process of acquiring SSI benefits was sometimes perceived as arbitrary and capricious and not readily subject to rational intervention, since key decisionmakers often could not be identified.

At the other extreme, some respondents reported that obtaining SSI assistance was a relatively smooth process that took about a month. They reported no particular problems and had a close working relationship with local social security office administrators. It is intriguing that both extremes existed in the same state.

Although the information collected in this study does not allow us to diagnose the nature of the problem with SSI, SSI was clearly a major source of concern for clients and staff. While SSI procedures may be sound but ineffectively implemented at the local level, there may also be some inherent problems with the procedures. Both the logic of the SSI system and its local administration should be carefully reviewed for their relationship to services for the mentally disabled.

Another problem related to SSI involved the procedures for establishing eligibility. These procedures included the necessity of filling out complex forms that clients had difficulty understanding or of providing supporting documents (birth certificates for example) that clients might not have. Some respondents indicated that the Social Security staff tended to be too busy to give the assistance that clients needed to negotiate these hurdles.

The uncertainty engendered by SSI is increased by regulations that withdraw support from clients who are rehospitalized, even for very brief periods. This procedure often caused clients to lose their community residences because they could not keep up their rent payments and produced another period of uncertainty while they tried to reestablish eligibility. A few respondents suggested that some SSI benefits should be made available to the rehospitalized patient so that dependence and uncertainty would be reduced.

Respondents also mentioned the additional cost of retaining clients in institutions while they awaited SSI eligibility determination, but they did not estimate the cost of prolonging institutional stays. At an average daily cost of $40 or $50, a delay of sixty to ninety days would appear to generate a sizable additional expenditure for institutional care. However, simple cost estimates are difficult to make because of fixed costs in institutional services and the inability to estimate the number of other clients who might be served if beds were vacated more quickly.

One state had instituted a procedure whereby clients could be released from institutions and supported from a revolving fund until SSI was obtained. A few respondents believed that the savings were well worth the unrecovered costs from clients who were eventually declared ineligible; but no analyses of actual savings were available.

It seems clear that SSI procedures had a negative impact on the quality of services clients received, as well as on their emotional stability. Problems in SSI procedures also appear to have caused cost increases. Without discarding necessary safeguards against abuse, SSI procedures should be simplified and expedited as much as possible. In addition, the threat of loss of eligibility should be minimized for individuals with established chronically disabling conditions.

While the comments of most respondents focused on the problems that SSI procedures created for clients, a significant problem for one state's administrative system also surfaced in discussions. When a client was sufficiently impaired to require a guardian to handle his or her financial affairs, the state reviewed potential guardians from among the client's relatives and friends and appointed one believed able to do a reasonable job. When the state judged either that there was no responsible relative or friend or that there would be a serious conflict of interest in appointing the available individual, one of the state's legal officers was appointed as the client's guardian. The Social Security Administration did not feel bound by this determination, however, and designated another guardian and sent the SSI payments to that individual. Thus, one person was legally designated by the state to be responsible for the client's financial affairs, but another individual was in control of what may be the client's main source of income. Some respondents reported that they had experienced instances in which the guardian appointed by SSI converted funds to his own uses and left the state's guardian without means to meet the client's obligations. A resolution between state and federal designation of a legal guardian for clients should be sought so that the same individual is selected by both.

Problems with Other Financial Assistance Programs

Forty-three percent of all respondents mentioned that they and their deinstitutionalized clients had experienced difficulties in obtaining public assistance and other sources of financial aid, such as food stamps and child welfare assistance. The complexity of the forms that must be completed, the variety of steps involved in the application process, and the delays in receiving benefits caused considerable frustration to staff members.

Problems in obtaining financial assistance were attributed to the fact that the state financial assistance staff did not necessarily view the mentally disabled as "their" clients but more appropriately as the clients of Social Security. The result was that clients often could not obtain a source of income quickly or that they stayed in institutions longer than necessary. In addition, monthly payments from state public assistance may be lower than SSI payments so that clients had to live in the worst housing and eat inadequately at a time that was particularly critical in terms of their community adjustment. Worry over unmet financial needs was said by some respondents to complicate clients' emotional problems. Staff frustration and negative impact on clients occurred because of delays and difficulties encountered when clients attempted to obtain various types of public assistance other than SSI. The operation of state and local financial assistance systems should be reviewed for possible changes to expedite the delivery of benefits to deinstitutionalized clients.

Conclusion

Funding patterns at both the federal and state levels caused considerable staff and client frustration. A number of the persons with whom discussions were held stated explicitly that funding patterns, rather than needs, seemed to control the services clients received. In addition, it was observed that a funding stream to support the objectives of deinstitutionalization was lacking. While Medicaid was seen as funding institutions and providing for clients' physical care, no adequate, equivalent stream to support community-based programs or clients' nonphysical needs was identified.

For this reason, we recommend that existing funding streams be reexamined for possible improvement in meeting this objective. In addition, policies should be devised for the development of support systems that have as their objective the maximization of each individual's self-sufficiency and the reduction of the dependency that often results from institutional-type care.

Social Issues

However commendable a change may be, the process of change disrupts established patterns and forces readjustments that are sometimes difficult for society to accept. The process of deinstitutionalization is such a change for both the members of a community and a client seeking placement in that community. This section discusses: (1) active opposition to deinstitutionalization by communities, and (2) other barriers that the client faced when placed in the community (see Table 4.3).

Community Opposition to Deinstitutionalized Clients

Concern for community acceptance of the mentally disabled was a major issue that was consistently mentioned by individuals at all levels within the mental health and mental retardation systems. Community opposition was discussed by 65 percent of all respondents. More specifically, the problems cited in community placement were: (1) negative attitudes, (2) zoning restrictions, and (3) oversaturation of neighborhoods.

Negative Attitudes. Forty-nine percent of all respondents felt that negative attitudes toward the mentally disabled were a

Table 4.3. SOCIAL ISSUES

	Discussed Issue	Percentage of all respondents (N=237) identifying problem
	N	%
Community Opposition	180	65
Negative Attitudes	134	49
Zoning	88	30
Oversaturation	56	23
Other Barriers		
Residential Alternatives	194	78
HUD Programs	43	16

problem and that these attitudes were due to a lack of awareness and understanding of client disabilities and needs. The community was said to be fearful and concerned about safety, possible negative influences of clients (particularly on children), and unattractive or odd behavior. The fear of violence on the part of clients was said to be particularly high following extensive media coverage of an incident in which a former client was involved. However, most respondents felt that the mentally disabled were more likely to be victims (rather than perpetrators) of criminal or aggressive behavior.

Some respondents were able to report incidents in which individuals who initially displayed negative attitudes toward clients later became their active supporters. This change in attitude was usually felt to be a function of direct, positive experiences with both clients and a supportive care-giving system. Thus, at least some of the public's poor image of the mentally disabled was a function of how responsibly the care-giving system supports clients and handles grievances.

Even among educated and generally sympathetic persons, fear and misunderstanding about the mentally disabled are common. However, negative attitudes can often be changed. Because consultation, education, and supportive activities on behalf of clients are not revenue-producing, they are highly vulnerable to budget cutbacks. Since unchallenged negative attitudes can easily thwart many of the positive effects of direct services, funding policies should include a contribution toward maintaining those services.

Zoning Restrictions. Negative attitudes and a lack of understanding of the mentally disabled have had a substantial impact on zoning ordinances and the establishment of community residential facilities. Problems with zoning restrictions were mentioned by 30 percent of all respondents. Neighborhoods were said to be concerned that: (1) allowing multiple resident homes in single family neighborhoods could trigger a change in the character of the neighborhood, (2) homes for the mentally disabled would degrade the peace and quiet of neighborhoods or cause increased traffic, and (3) property values would decline. However, a few persons thought property values might rise because homes would be renovated and yards would be cared for as some made an effort to be "good neighbors."

When invoked, zoning was a potent impediment to developing community placements in certain neighborhoods. While some respondents reported successes in defeating such blocks, many felt that it was better to develop placements in more receptive parts of the community. Some felt "caught in the middle" between recognizing the legitimate right of communities to determine their own character and the rights of the mentally disabled to live in nonrestrictive and appropriate community surroundings. Several persons suggested that the right of mentally disabled clients to live in communities was constitutionally guaranteed and could be reinforced through government funding policies. At least one respondent suggested that federal funds not be distributed to localities that could not provide evidence of nondiscrimination against the mentally handicapped.

The right of the mentally disabled to live in the community should be clearly established by public policy. Negotiations should focus on the areas within the community that would best meet the needs of both residents and mentally disabled clients.

Oversaturation of Neighborhoods. Twenty-three percent of all respondents indicated that communities were concerned about the possibility that an extremely high concentration of mentally disabled persons would settle in their areas. Because of such factors as uneven placement, zoning restrictions, the availability or lack of suitable housing, or proximity to institutions, some neighborhoods had absorbed particularly high concentrations of deinstitutionalized clients. Some of these neighborhoods were old and decaying and were densely populated, with low income residents; some were largely commercial; some were older, hotel districts; and some were inhabited by poor residents, who were unable to politically oppose the residential placement of the mentally disabled. The concern about oversaturation was so great in one county that a saturation index, which was used to guide planning for new community placement, had been developed.

Some of the opposition to over-concentrating clients in certain areas was economic in nature. In some states, localities had to cover part of the costs of keeping clients. Counties that contained state hospitals or schools for the retarded often absorbed a high proportion of deinstitutionalized clients simply because of convenience and proximity. Thus, host counties may have ended up supporting many clients who were not originally their residents. In some cases these areas have responded by resisting additional placements. An objective index of saturation should be adopted for monitoring and planning the deinstitutionalization process to make sure that localities are accepting their share of the responsibility for the deinstitutionalized population.

Other Barriers to Placing Deinstitutionalized Clients in the Community

Lack of Residential Alternatives. Deinstitutionalization involves more than the simple movement of individuals out of institutions. An important element of this process is placing individuals in the most appropriate and least restrictive residential alternatives and gradually involving them in the community.

Seventy-eight percent of all individuals with whom discussions were held agreed that there was a clear need for better quality, a wider range, and a larger number of community residential facilities. In almost every case, respondents mentioned that they were aware that specific alternatives, which they either knew existed elsewhere or could easily imagine, would be desirable in their areas. Specifically, they stated there was a need for: (1) more family-oriented residential settings, such as group homes, foster homes, and respite care facilities; and (2) more transitional programs that provided less supervision than insitutions but greater supervision than independent living arrangements. Essentially, respondents were interested in developing a full range of residential placement in order to best accomodate the varying needs of clients. Moreover, they wished to have the flexibility to offer clients an opportunity to change their living arrangements as their needs changed.

However, funding was a barrier in many cases, since the existing residential arrangement tended to be linked to some stream of funding, and developing alternative residential arrangements would require additional funding streams. In other cases, the issue was not how to find a funding stream but how to get "front-end" money to develop the desired alternatives. Sometimes individuals were required to develop residences that met certain standards and then demonstrate their operation for six months before they could become eligible for payments. Sometimes simply meeting fire and building codes required by Medicaid and HUD was out of the financial reach of most potential operators of residential programs.

Thus, funding tends to be linked to specific kinds of residential arrangements rather than to client needs. Without the flexibility to place and move clients as their needs or preferences dictated, providers were constantly in the position of placing clients in facilities that happened to be available rather than in facilities best suited to their clients' needs. Within reasonable financial limits, the widest possible range of residential arrangements should be made available to clients based on their needs, rather than on funding considerations.

Difficulties with HUD Programs. One potential major source of funds for housing alternatives is the Section 8 Housing Assistance Payments Program that is part of the Housing and Community Development Act (P.L. 93-383) administered by the Department of Housing and Urban Development (HUD). Under this program an individual who is defined as handicapped and is in the low-income bracket can qualify for a rental subsidy in rehabilitated, new, or existing housing.

Although relatively few respondents mentioned that they had attempted to use the HUD program, 16 percent of the total number of respondents viewed it as very complex and difficult to interface with. Many persons stated that filling out HUD forms was a task that only a full-time person or a knowledgeable consultant should undertake. One respondent suggested that because of the high cost of applying for money to build community residences, special funding should be provided to cover the cost of interacting with HUD. Thus, while a few successful encounters with HUD were described, the overall impression was that the HUD program did not help deinstitutionalized individuals because it was too difficult, time consuming, and costly to access.

HUD programs should be reviewed with representatives of the care-giving system to find ways to make them more accessible. A potential conflict between HUD and the Social Security Administration (SSA) in determining if SSI beneficiaries can maintain their benefits while receiving HUD assistance should also be reviewed.

Conclusion

Persons with whom discussions were held noted three major barriers to the community placement of deinstitutionalized clients: (1) the community's unwillingness to accept clients, (2) the lack of an adequate range of residential alternatives in the community, and (3) the difficulties involved in using HUD rental subsidies to house clients. All of these problems make the deinstitutionalization movement's goal of placing clients in the least restrictive and most appropriate environment possible very difficult to achieve.

The attempt to exclude and restrict the mentally disabled from community settings is not a recent development. Since the nineteenth century, society has attempted to isolate these persons. At present, negative attitudes and exclusionary tendencies are being expressed through zoning restrictions in some areas, which lead to oversaturation of clients in other areas. The possible decline of property values is also used to justify exclusion.

Opposition to the placement of deinstitutionalized clients in community settings has negatively affected clients, frustrated system staff and policymakers, and increased the cost of care. Many clients remain in institutions simply because they lack residential alternatives, and others have been placed in poor housing in run-down neighborhoods, so that the process of normalization has, in effect, been slowed. Finally, when clients remain in institutions unnecessarily, costs certainly increase.

In addition, because of the difficulties involved in funding the development of residential alternatives, many clients must be placed in facilities that are inappropriate for their needs. Inappropriate or delayed placements have a negative impact on both clients and staff.

Because of the significant barriers posed by negative attitudes and the lack of a funding stream, more attempts should be funded both to educate and negotiate with the communities where clients are placed. Saturation indices may be useful to avoid community opposition and relieve unfounded fears of oversaturation. Finally, a reassessment and simplification of the HUD application process may be in order.

Other Significant Issues

Although most of the persons with whom discussions were held concentrated their remarks on the three areas mentioned previously, a number of respondents discussed other issues that they felt influenced the way in which the deinstitutionalization effort has been implemented. Their remarks focused primarily on (1) the difficulty of balancing the rights of clients and of the community, (2) the barrier to continuity of care posed by confidentiality of information requirements in some states, and (3) the importance of training and improving working conditions within community care facilities.

The Rights of Clients Versus the Rights of the Community

Respondents frequently discussed the difficulty of effectively balancing clients' needs for treatment in the least restrictive settings possible (which frequently meant treatment in the community) with the community's need for protection from persons who were possibly dangerous. Legal decisions that have reinforced clients' rights and have sought to protect clients from arbitrary confinement have also generally limited the conditions under which clients may be institutionalized; there are three such conditions: (1) the patient is a danger to himself/herself, (2) the patient is a danger to others, or (3) the patient is too gravely impaired to manage his or her own affairs.

Even though these provisions are designed to protect clients, a few respondents expressed concern that, in some cases, they also worked to the clients' detriment. If clients did not agree to continue treatment voluntarily after initial involuntary commitment, staff frequently discharged them into the community rather than go through the complex and time-consuming process of seeking long-term involuntary commitment. Some persons who had only been partially treated were, therefore, released. The likelihood that such people would return to the institution was said to be high.

In addition, a few respondents mentioned cases in which persons who had been released prematurely from institutions committed suicide or harmed others. These incidents were covered in the media and, although they were generally the exception rather than the rule, they reinforced community opposition to the deinstitutionalization process.

One of the objectives of the deinstitutionalization process was to create a more equitable balance between the rights of the client and of the community. Previously the community's need for protection usually took precedence over the client's constitutional rights. Although some respondents felt that the attempt to remedy this situation had been carried too far, most were still concerned with protecting clients' rights. However, they felt that this objective had not necessarily been furthered by currently tight legal requirements for involuntary commitment.

Confidentiality Requirements

The rules governing the handling of confidential client information have also been tightened, again in response to past abuses. One of the most troublesome and expensive steps in serving a client is gathering the evaluation and background information needed to plan treatment. However, in spite of the emphasis on the integration of services and interagency cooperation, some respondents reported that they were often unable to obtain needed client information from other agencies because of confidentiality regulations. These regulations resulted in delays in providing services or expensive, duplicative regathering of information. In some cases these requirements meant that continuity of treatment was not possible. Although respondents did not object to confidentiality requirements, they did question the extent of such safeguards.

The Need for Staff Training

Respondents frequently mentioned the important role of training in improving the operation of the deinstitutionalization process. Providing basic training in the nature of various mental disabilities and the best methods of dealing with these disabilities was seen as central in strengthening community-based care. Many respondents emphasized the necessity of providing nursing home and boarding home staff with such training. However, they lamented the fact that even when such training was available it often had little, if any, effect. Because of low wages and heavy responsibilities, staff members rarely stayed in their jobs long enough to apply newly acquired skills.

The importance of retraining institutional staff was also emphasized by respondents. Many attitudes conveyed to clients in institutions were said to be inappropriate in community settings, and many jobs in institutional facilities have no equivalents in community care systems. Thus, preparing employees to take on new responsibilities and to relate to clients in new ways is critical. Providing incentives for institutional employees to relocate and for urban professional staff to move to rural areas was also suggested by several respondents.

Conclusion

The conflict involved in providing the best treatment for clients and protecting their constitutional rights through involuntary treatment acts and confidentiality requirements while simultaneously safeguarding the community has caused considerable difficulty for some elements of the care-giving system. While originally intended to remedy past abuses and violations of clients' rights, legal regulations today often make it difficult to completely treat mentally ill persons. Little is currently known about the specific impact and implications of recent legal decisions on clients, staff, the care-giving system, and the community.

Training, retraining, and relocating employees were also mentioned as significant issues. All were seen as necessary to improve the operation of the deinstitutionalization process, to meet client needs, and to reduce resistance to the process from within the system.

An illustration of the etiology and possible extent of the problem appears in Figures 4.1–4.6. Figure 4.1 describes the variety of ways in which a patient can be discharged. Figures 4.2–4.5 detail the implications for each of the possible discharge considerations. For Figures 4.2 through 4.5, it should be noted that all categories to the right of the column labeled "Possible Discharge Considerations" represent potential options and that these options are not displayed in any particular order. That is, a person is just as likely to be discharged to any one of the options as another. Finally, Figure 4.6 provides "A Random Walk Through the Deinstitutionalization Process" and details the possible consequences of a discharge decision.

Delays in receiving SSI may also have significantly increased costs to the system. When clients remained in institutional settings unnecessarily, cost-effectiveness was certainly reduced. In addition, if hospital beds were in short supply, other patients who needed in-hospital care may not have been able to receive it.

Because the care-giving system extracts a significant toll on the effectiveness and efficiency of the personnel in the system, there should be an inquiry into the effects of administrative controls and incentive systems on the effectiveness and efficiency of staff. An effort should be made to quantify these effects so that the costs and benefits can be compared.

Impact of Problems with the Deinstitutionalization Process

A large number of persons with whom discussions were held stated that the way in which deinstitutionalization has been carried out has caused further difficulties for clients who were already handicapped in several ways and has also had a negative effect on staffs and the care-giving system.

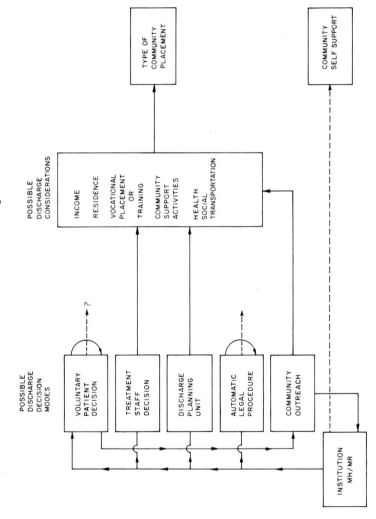

FIGURE 4.1
Deinstitutionalization Discharge Decision

FIGURE 4.2

Possible Discharge Considerations—Income

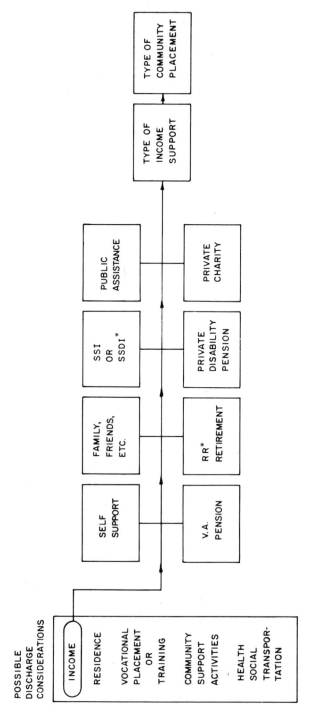

*Social Security Disability Insurance

**Railroad

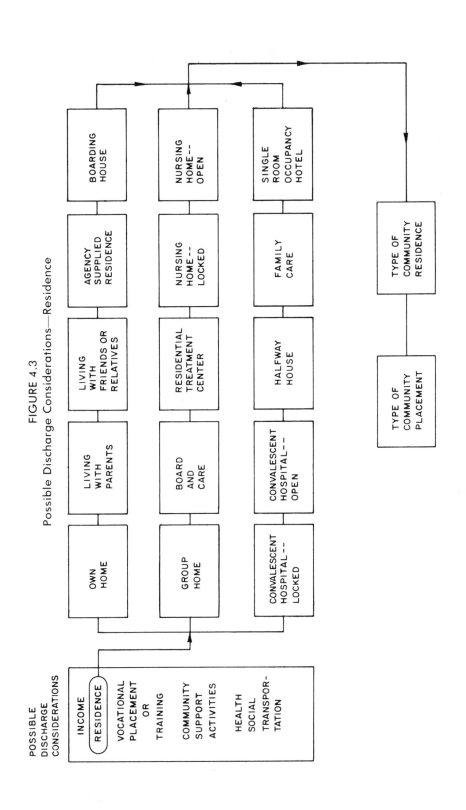

FIGURE 4.3
Possible Discharge Considerations—Residence

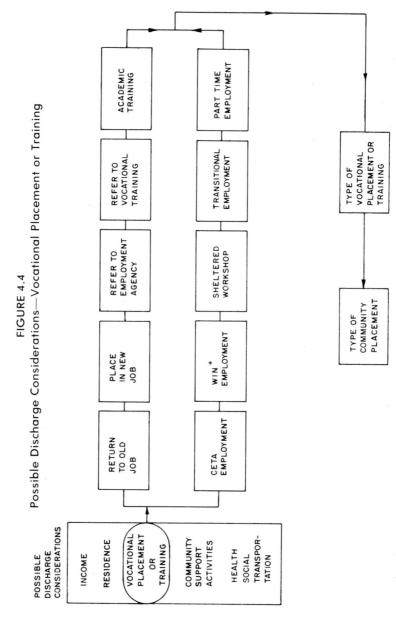

FIGURE 4.4

Possible Discharge Considerations—Vocational Placement or Training

*Work Incentive Program

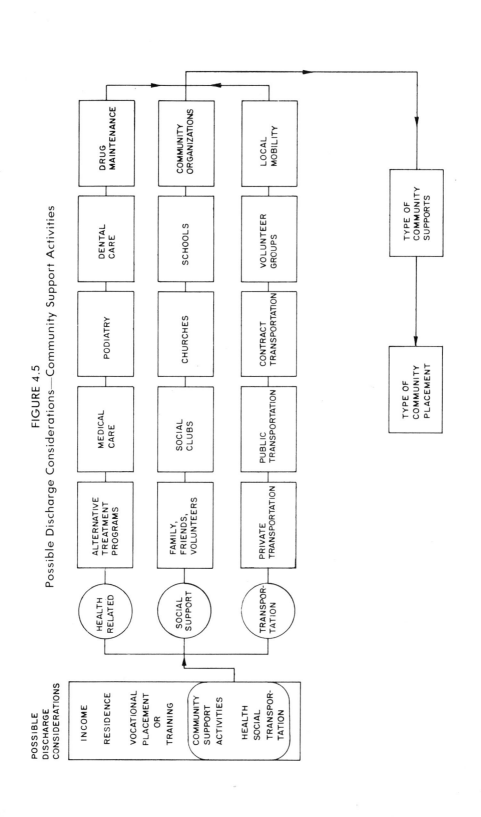

FIGURE 4.5
Possible Discharge Considerations—Community Support Activities

FIGURE 4.6

A Random Walk Through the Deinstitutionalization Process

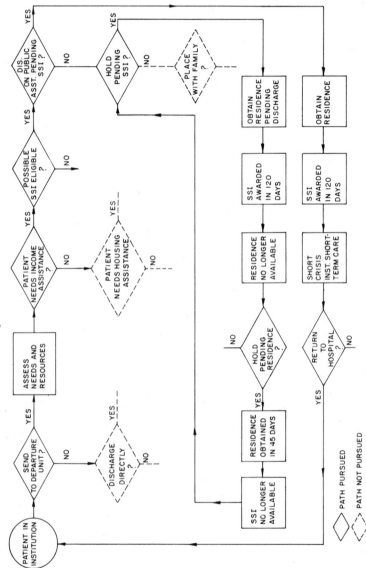

Impact on Clients

The main concern of this research project was that the process of deinstitutionalization was not going well for many clients. Although a number of the barriers and problems that have accompanied the deinstitutionalization process have been identified by past studies, little systematic attention has been focused upon the impact these problems have on clients. Thus, a major purpose of this study was to attempt to determine the negative impact on clients, if any, of specific aspects of the deinstitutionalization process (see Table 4.4).

Many respondents were administrators who did not deliver direct services and thus did not have occasion to directly observe client reactions. However, a majority of those respondents who did observe clients directly or who had extensive second-hand knowledge of clients through supervision or other administrative relationships (68 percent) agreed that the fragmentation of the care-giving system and the process by which deinstitutionalization has occurred have had a negative impact on clients. More specifically, 40 percent of all respondents stated that mentally ill and mentally retarded clients experienced increased confusion, agitation, depression and boredom, that levels of antisocial behavior and victimization rose, and that greater neglect of physical needs

Table 4.4. IMPACTS ON CLIENTS

	Discussed Issue	Percentage of all respondents (N=237) identifying problem
	N	%
Negative Impacts	165	68
Negative Emotions	99	40
Physical Neglect	61	24
Return to Institution	112	47
More Restrictive Environment	88	37
Antisocial Behavior	58	24
Victimization	13	5

was apparent because of the nature of the deinstitutionalization process. In addition, certain aspects of the deinstitutionalization process were said to result in greater disruptions
of the lives of clients and their families. Ironically, the process itself was frequently observed to result in the placement
of clients in environments that were more restrictive than
necessary or even to lead to prolonged stays in or readmit-
tance to institutions. Clearly, one of the major objectives of
the process of deinstitutionalization – to improve the quality
of life and to maximize the opportunities and self-sufficiency
of clients within the least restrictive settings possible – is not
being met.

Several aspects of the process were said to contribute to
these problems. Respondents spoke of delays in finding community placements for clients who had been prepared for
discharge and who had progressively moved into more independent settings within institutions. In addition, they
stated that the failure to obtain timely financial assistance
caused delays in leaving institutions and contributed to
greater client difficulty in the community. Prolonging institutional stays may be especially damaging when clients have
been psychologically prepared to leave institutions. Even if
state assistance was obtained, clients were still vulnerable
because they received checks that were smaller than the pro-
mised SSI checks. Yet their first checks probably determined
where they would be able to live. Thus, delays forced clients
to locate in the worst neighborhoods.

As a result of the difficulty in obtaining SSI, some clients
became very reluctant to endanger their eligibility by earning
too much money. They knew they might function well
enough to hold a job for a while, but they also knew that their
problems were recurring. Although clients knew that they
would probably require SSI support again, they feared that
they might not be able to obtain it the next time they needed
it. Hence, a procedure designed to prevent people from getting on the SSI roles unnecessarily also worked to keep them

on those roles once they received SSI. Further, this obstacle to work helped defeat one of the major goals for many of these clients: providing them with both the satisfaction and income from productive activity.

Some respondents stated that clients were leaving institutions so quickly that they were not adequately treated before they left and there was not time to plan a community placement for them. A few operators of community facilities complained that mental patients arrived too disturbed to function in their setting and rapidly deteriorated to the point of needing rehospitalization. This was harmful to the clients, and it was distressing to other clients living in these settings.

Boredom, frustration, and self-doubt increased when clients could not be placed in vocational rehabilitation/vocational training programs, sheltered workshops, or jobs. Delays were frequently experienced because placements were unavailable, clients were not enthusiastic about the choices available to them, or vocational programs and the staffs of such programs were not geared toward dealing with deinstitutionalized clients. Clients' senses of self-worth were often said to be linked to involvement in work activities. Many who worked with the retarded stated that unstructured time was particularly difficult for their clients to deal with.

Finally, respondents stated that the lack of adequate recreational and socialization activities in the community caused clients difficulties. While respondents noted that because of this lack some clients wished to return to institutions, the majority of clients were reported to prefer noninstitutional life, despite its hardships.

Many respondents described increases in antisocial behavior, victimization, and neglect of physical needs as negative impacts of the deinstitutionalization process. Twenty-four percent of the respondents stated that the mentally ill, and to a lesser degree the retarded, neglected their physical needs because of the lack of adequate follow-up and outreach services and very low income levels. Some persons observed that clients sometimes stopped taking their medications, preferring to use what little money they had for other activities, such as entertainment. Clients also neglected their needs for medical and dental care. The nature of their mental illness or retardation made them unaware or incapable of recognizing medical or dental needs or insufficiently motivated or capable of aggressively seeking out this help on their own.

As a result of antisocial behavior and/or going off of medications, some clients returned to institutions or were placed in more restrictive environments. Forty-seven percent of those with whom discussions were held observed that clients returned to institutions because of problems in the deinstitutionalization process, and 37 percent noted that they ended up in more restrictive environments than were necessary because of these problems. A client who exhibited violent or antisocial behavior that often resulted from medication problems frequently had to be returned to an institution because of a lack of acute inpatient facilities or the resistance of private hospitals to taking psychiatric patients. Even if acute facilities were available, recycling into inpatient status was likely to occur because the problems clients faced (lack of outreach services, for example) continued to exist. Some respondents noted that retarded and elderly clients attempted to return to institutions because they had more access to recreational activities there than they did in the community. For others, the simple assurance of access to food and clothing in the institution made it an attractive alternative.

Twenty-four percent of all respondents observed that antisocial behavior occurred as a result of certain aspects of the deinstitutionalization process, and a few persons (5 percent) discussed the occurrence of victimization. Reasons given for these problems included the existence of unstructured time and residential placement in poorer neighborhoods where criminal elements resided. The presence of negative role models, the lack of peer group social support from other sources, and the lack of living skills training (for example, money management) were seen as contributing to unacceptable behavior and victimization.

Finally, a number of persons indicated that institutional staff resistance to deinstitutionalization negatively affected clients' chances of successfully adjusting to life in the community. This resistance was said to affect clients primarily in two ways. First, those being readied for discharge were likely to receive the message, either overtly or covertly, that they were not expected to "make it" on the outside. Some persons complained that institutional staff had not adequately prepared clients for discharge, thereby setting into motion a self-fulfilling prophecy. Second, in an effort to find alternative employment, some institutional staff members were encouraged to become proprietors of family care or board and care homes. A few respondents reported that some former institutional employees continued to treat clients in a dependency-inducing manner and did not encourage them to make use of community resources.

Therefore, the mere creation of community alternatives does not necessarily ensure that a self-sufficiency–oriented care philosophy will be practiced. Community placements can become "mini-insitutions," practicing a custodial, dependency-inducing philosophy, rather than fostering treatment and the maximization of self-sufficiency.

It is clear that placement in the community exposed clients to a wide variety of hazards and resulted in many significant physical and mental problems. In spite of these drawbacks, community placement was generally preferred by clients. There should be a regular and systematic monitoring of community adjustment of clients by specifically designated elements within the care-giving system.

Impact on Staffs and the System

While the major focus of this study was the impact of the

deinstitutionalization process on clients, a number of negative impacts on staffs and the care-giving system were also
found to exist. Much energy was tied up and much frustration was generated by the way the system operated. Frustra-
tions that clients endured once, staffs were subject to day
after day. This frustration translated directly into lowered
staff productivity and increased administrative overhead.
Several respondents suggested that frustration with the
system was a greater source of staff "burn out" than the task
of working with difficult people who have difficult problems.

For example, delays in receiving SSI exerted a negative impact on staff. A staff member may have found a residence for
a person, expecting that their SSI eligibility would be obtained on a certain date, thus enabling them to get a check
from public welfare. If eligibility was not obtained, the
residency might be lost. Thus, clients ended up in less appropriate residential facilities than were once available,
which may eventually discourage staff members from even
seeking out the most appropriate alternatives. In addition,
they often witnessed clients regressing while they waited for
benefits; renewed treatment was necessary.

Conclusion

Respondents stated that the process of deinstitutionalization resulted in negative impacts on clients, staffs, and the
care-giving system. Clients who experienced prolonged stays
in institutions because of delays in receiving financial assistance or obtaining suitable housing were said to have experienced increased frustration and frequent regression, which
often resulted in their returning to the institution. Clients also
experienced difficulties in obtaining vocational and recreational opportunities, which raised their level of boredom and
self-doubt and sometimes led to involvement in illegal or antisocial activities.

Members of the care-giving staff and the system as a whole
were also negatively affected by the process. Frustration was

said to result in lowered productivity and eventual "burn out." System costs increased when clients were maintained in more restrictive settings and had to be returned to institutions because of negative experiences in the community.

Greater attention should be paid to the negative impact of the deinstitutionalization process on clients, staffs, and the system. Specific causes and effects of the process and the costs and benefits of certain practices should be quantified.

5
Summary and Implications of the Results

This study was designed to identify problems related to the care-giving system and the process of deinstitutionalization. Open-ended discussions with 279 respondents clearly revealed that negative impacts on clients, staffs, and the care-giving system have resulted from the way in which the deinstitutionalization effort has been implemented. Each of the four problem areas that were identified created difficulties for staffs and for clients attempting to adapt to community settings.

Problem Areas

Problems in defining agency and staff roles and responsibilities, opposition to deinstitutionalization from within the political and care-giving systems, and difficulties in accessing the generic services needed by clients produced a number of negative impacts on clients. Where responsibilities for aftercare services and multidiagnosis clients were unclear, clients were frequently shuffled among various elements of the system or they fell between the cracks until a crisis occurred, at which time they might be transferred to a state hospital or some other restrictive setting, such as a jail.

In addition, opposition to deinstitutionalization by some of the care-giving staff members gave some clients an implicit message that they were not expected to survive in the com-

munity. Other staff members may have unintentionally encouraged client dependence. Still others neglected the needs
of chronic patients, with the result that these clients often
returned to institutions or somehow survived without access
to treatment. Opposition to deinstitutionalization by many
families and communities also limited clients' opportunities
to live in the least restrictive setting possible.

The complexities of using generic services posed considerable problems for both clients and staffs. One respondent observed that if clients were strong enough to successfully negotiate the service system, they would be healthy
enough not to need it. Other respondents described the
frustration they experienced in attempting to help clients use
these services.

Economic or cost-related issues were another source of difficulty. Since funding patterns rather than client needs determined the services, clients were frequently placed in residential facilities that were more restrictive than would have been
ideal. The failure to deliver appropriate services was said by
some respondents to have resulted in regression or greater
client dependency.

Many clients also experienced frustration in the process of
trying to obtain financial assistance. When this assistance
was not provided in a timely manner, clients often had to remain in institutions longer than necessary and many regressed. Those who were released frequently had difficulty
in locating housing because of delays in receiving SSI. For
many clients, the first month out of the institution was
especially critical, and it was during this time that they had
the least financial resources.

Clients also experienced frustration when they sought
residence in the community. Negative community attitudes
toward clients, which were often expressed through zoning
restrictions and by expressions of fear that neighborhoods
would be oversaturated, made it difficult to place clients in
many areas. Clients, therefore, often ended up living in less

desirable but more accepting neighborhoods, which were commercial, decaying, or possibly unsafe. Normalization was virtually impossible in such settings.

In addition, clients were often not placed in the most appropriate or least restrictive residential settings because potential operators could not obtain front-end money for their development and could not meet strict building and fire codes and high continuation costs. HUD funds were so difficult to access that many staff respondents were discouraged after trying to use them and many more may not have tried to do so. The result, once again, was that clients took up residence in available facilities rather than in the facilities that best met their needs.

Although recent legal decisions have corrected many past abuses of clients' constitutional rights, they have also created problems for clients and staffs. Stringent standards for obtaining involuntary commitments often mean that some patients who needed long-term institutional care are released although they may be a danger to the community or themselves. Sometimes these clients have to be rehospitalized. Although staff members often spent long hours at legal hearings, some felt that their views were not adequately considered.

Requirements concerning confidentiality of information, while protecting client rights, made it difficult for staffs to provide continuous treatment for clients released from institutions. Medication routines were sometimes interrupted or changed when records were not available, and some clients regressed and had to return to institutions.

As was stated in Chapter 2, the objectives of deinstitutionalization are: (1) to provide treatment for clients in the least restrictive settings possible, (2) to provide this treatment at the lowest possible cost, and (3) to provide clients with supportive services. In other words, the overriding purpose of deinstitutionalization might be said to be maximizing individuals' self-sufficiency while recognizing the existence of resource limitations and societal rights.

The results of this study indicated that the overall objectives of the deinstitutionalization effort had not been met. More specifically, clients had not been placed in the least restrictive care environments because certain current funding patterns were inconsistent with the objectives of the movement. Similarly, costs had not been reduced. When clients were forced to remain in institutions – because of delays in receiving financial assistance, a lack of community residential alternatives, and community opposition to their release – or were placed in more expensive and restrictive settings than they needed because they had nowhere else to go, costs of care increased. Finally, supportive services were often unavailable because of the inaccessibility of many generic services and a lack of clear responsibility for outreach and follow-up services.

Although these problems are complex and serious, many can be at least partially solved within the current system. However, if the system as it presently operates is allowed to continue, then a variety of negative outcomes may endanger the deinstitutionalization effort.

More specifically, the backlash against placement of the mentally disabled in communities will almost certainly continue and/or become worse. If no aggressive action is taken by way of education or legal pressure, there will also be a decline in the development of more appropriate and less restrictive community services, which are only now starting in many areas. In places where opposition has already occurred, many people have been placed in restrictive, mini-institutional settings such as nursing homes and developmental centers for the mentally retarded; or, in some instances, patients remained in institutions longer than necessary or ended up in the worst neighborhoods. Ghettoization is certainly not a positive move in the direction of normalization in the community. If many of these problems are not solved, we will see the development of more mini-institutions, more shuffling of people from one institutional setting to another, and more movement from the back wards of institutions to the back alleys of communities. The development of mini-institutions may lead both the public and policymakers to reconsider the value of the deinstitutionalization effort and to plan new alternatives. Thus, we urge that the movement toward deinstitutionalization not be taken for granted. Although its problems are multiple and significant, it can be improved.

Positive Results

In spite of the complexity and severity of some of the problems that have been discussed, the deinstitutionalization process has resulted in some positive outcomes. Some respondents mentioned the increase in citizen involvement and the growth of advocacy and volunteer groups that provided needed social support to the mentally disabled who were attempting to adjust to community life. While this study has indicated that much remains to be done to quiet community opposition to deinstitutionalization efforts, a considerable enlightenment of the public does appear to have occurred in the past two decades.

Respondents pointed to additional positive results. First, innovative social programs in the community sector have been developed. Second, there have also been some improvements in the conditions in many institutions: state facilities are less crowded; in many places client/staff ratios have improved; and institutions have broadened their functions.

It was also apparent from our discussions that, even though respondents were often frustrated with the difficulties involved in attempting to implement the deinstitutionalization ideology, only a very few would have argued against the continuation of the effort. While individuals differed on specifics – the most appropriate timing for the effort, the problems posed by funding levels, and the future role of institutions, for example – most agreed that clients could and should be helped to become as self-sufficient as possible in the community if the proper mechanisms were available. Almost everyone with whom we met, including institutional employees, stressed that the welfare of clients was primary; they focused criticism on some of the poorly planned and executed efforts at deinstitutionalization in the past.

In addition, virtually no one argued against the deinstitutionalization philosophy. Many staff members and policymakers were simply frustrated with the barriers to its implementation and the complexity of the current system. Most respondents clearly understood the problems they faced, but, given their complexity, they did not know how to tackle them effectively. Yet, in spite of the difficulties of operating within a fragmented system with inadequate resources, they were still willing to expend a great deal of energy to develop and improve programs for clients.

Areas for Improvement

Specifically, respondents described four major areas that needed attention: (1) problems in establishing a stable source of income for clients, (2) barriers to accessing a wide range of appropriate residential and supportive services, (3) problems in reaching a better balance between client and community rights, and (4) difficulties in establishing a nondependency-inducing support system.

1. A stable and adequate source of income is necessary if the chronically disabled are to survive in the community. Although the SSI system was the greatest source of that income, it was also a major source of distress. Reviewing and modifying the operations of the SSI system should be a top priority in improving the deinstitutionalization process.

2. A great deal could be done with existing technology to maximize the productivity and self-sufficiency of the chroni-

cally disabled. Barriers to the achievement of this objective were described as mostly administrative and financial. Although in many communities services are available, coordinating mechanisms must be developed so that clients can easily take advantage of these services. A number of respondents mentioned that the development of adequately funded case management systems could provide this coordination. Respondents also stated that funding patterns should be reviewed and changed so that the services clients received would be dictated by their needs. System incentives, particularly for mental health centers and other community-based services, were also seen as necessary if clients were to use the services that they needed.

3. The care-giving system is still adjusting to the increased protection that recent legal decisions have given to clients. Involuntary admissions are severely limited; clients must be treated in the least restrictive environment; and confidentiality of client information is strongly protected. While supporting the intent of all these safeguards, respondents feared that as these safeguards were currently being applied they were serving neither the best interests of the client nor the best interests of the community. Because it was anticipated that the legal system would play an increasingly important role in relation to the care-giving system, it was considered urgent that a constructive review of present and future interactions be undertaken.

4. While access to needed services can make the chronically disabled individual's life more productive, the ways in which these services are delivered can determine greater or lesser degrees of self-sufficiency. Respondents noted that not only were clients being moved from institutions to the community, but the custodial philosophy was also being exported. Respondents indicated an urgent need for the further development of community support systems that tend to move people to greater self-sufficiency, rather than institutional-type community systems where incentives favor con-

tinued client dependency.

These four issues represent the most pressing concerns with which the deinstitutionalization effort must deal if it is to continue. Although the problems are complex, they can be lessened or even corrected. Chapter 6 identifies a number of policy changes that can be made within the current system to improve the deinstitutionalization effort. In addition, it deals with the need to examine alternative systems that might alleviate or correct current problems.

Differences Between Mental Health and Mental Retardation Programs

The problems that accompany the deinstitutionalization process can be understood as part and parcel of an exceedingly diversified and complex political and human services care-giving network. From the discussions with individuals in the mental health and mental retardation fields, it was apparent that workers in both areas encountered many of the same problems, such as the inadequate delivery of community services, confusion and fragmentation of staff roles and responsibilities, competition for funds, coordination of treatment for the multidiagnosis client, and vocational placement and training. On the other hand, mental health and mental retardation professionals had very different problems and concerns in four areas: (1) differences in state mental health and mental retardation programs; (2) differences in the development and support of community-based programs; (3) differences in federal programs and eligibility requirements; and (4) differences in income maintenance.

Factors Influencing Variations Between State Mental Health and Mental Retardation Programs

As was expected, the states selected for the study varied in the degree to which they had developed and maintained programs for the mentally ill and mentally retarded. Some of the differences were obvious in the states' mental health and developmental disabilities programs. Other differences were identified during the site visits. For example, it was found that one state heavily supported its mental health programs (both institutional and community), while the state's developmental disabilities system struggled for visibility. On the other hand, other states had extensively developed systems for providing community-based services to the mentally retarded. Furthermore, the funding available to programs designed to serve the developmentally disabled was far in excess of that available for mental health community-based treatment.

There may be several factors that contributed to this disparity, including administrators' perceptions of the state's needs and interests, funding competition, and availability of qualified and effective professional staff members. However, the most important factor distinguishing programs for the mentally ill from programs for the mentally retarded was the existence of a set of well-organized advocacy groups. Advocacy groups (which may include lobbyists, state associations for the mentally retarded or mentally ill, and citizen advisory committees) have demonstrated their effectiveness in making the system respond to the client's views of his or her interests and needs. In the past, advocacy groups have also been very influential in demanding and monitoring the provision of community-based services and the rights of individuals residing in institutions.

At present, federal legislation mandates the provision of an advocacy system for the developmentally disabled (Developmental Disabilities Act of 1975). However, this system applies only to the developmentally disabled, not to the mentally ill. Although the Community Mental Health Center Act authorizes funding for advocacy projects, such funds are rarely, if ever, used. In March of 1978 legislation was introduced into Congress (S. 2722) emphasizing statewide advocacy for the mentally ill population. The bill was not passed into law, however, and from a national perspective it is clear that the mentally retarded and developmentally disabled are in a much stronger position (legally, politically, and financially) to support the development and maintenance of community based services.

A critical issue with regard to deinstitutionalization of either the mentally ill or the mentally retarded was the degree to which the availability of programs varied *within* a state. For instance, states that emphasized programs for the mentally retarded were more likely to have the political and financial resources needed for effectively implementing the goals of deinstitutionalization. Likewise, in states where programs for the mentally ill were better developed, mental health deinstitutionalization processes were also better developed.

Perhaps more important than the existence of advocacy groups and the availability of programs was the fact that rarely are "all things equal." In general, many factors identified as barriers to deinstitutionalization were less of a problem for the mentally retarded than the mentally ill. These problems and barriers are discussed in detail in the following sections.

Variations in the Development and Support
of Community Programs

The development and maintenance of community-based services was clearly a concern of both the mental health and developmental disabilities systems. However, individuals in the mental retardation system repeatedly raised the issue of coordinating services and facilities at the community level. Again, the severity of this problem varied from state to state. Nevertheless, the inflexibility and independence of local agencies serving the mentally retarded was discussed quite frequently. For example, workers in states with an extensive system for serving the mentally retarded mentioned that although the full range of services existed at the local level, there were barriers to influencing, coordinating, and monitoring local agencies and facilities. Moreover, many agencies were reluctant to support deinstitutionalization efforts, and, in many instances, no one had the authority to enforce or require the agency's cooperation.

On the other hand, states that did not emphasize mental retardation programs experienced additional problems in developing community-based programs. The problems included shortages in the types of programs needed and instability and temporary existence of residential facilities – all of which are obstacles to the deinstitutionalization effort. Perhaps the lack of coordination and fragmentation of community services contributed to resistance on the part of parents of the mentally retarded, institutions, and a few advocacy groups. Although members of both the mental health and mental retardation systems expressed varying degrees of resistance to deinstitutionalization, workers in the mental retardation system expressed more vociferously their belief that deinstitutionalization for the severely mentally retarded would not occur until adequate services and facilities existed in the community.

The difficulties resulting from fragmented services and lack of *local* coordination was cited less often by personnel in the mental health system. This situation may be attributed to the existence of community mental health centers that were established to coordinate community services for the mentally ill. At present, most state developmental disabilities systems do not have the authority, funding, or resources needed for coordinating and administering local services for the mentally retarded.

It appeared that community attitude toward the mentally retarded was generally more positive than toward the mentally ill. Residents perceived the mentally ill as a greater threat to personal safety, as more violent, and as less acceptable to the community than the mentally retarded. This attitude was partly the result of the media's coverage and criticism of the practice described as "dumping [the mentally ill] into the streets." As a result, the mental health system faced the oversaturation of the mentally ill in urban areas and zoning ordinances that restricted the mentally ill from residing in certain residential areas. In some states, mentally retarded clients might have been confronted with the same obstacles; however, perhaps due to recent legislation forbidding discrimination against the developmentally disabled and the existence of strong advocacy and parent groups, the general public seemed to be more aware of the barriers facing and the facts concerning the mentally retarded than those of the mentally ill. Consequently, community resistance to bringing the mentally disabled into the mainstream of community life appeared to be more of a struggle for the mentally ill than it was for the mentally retarded.

Differences in Federal Programs
and Eligibility Requirements

There are several federally initiated programs that are directed toward the mentally retarded for which the mentally ill do not qualify. Some of these programs are mandated by federal legislation (for example, the Developmental Disabilities Act, The Rehabilitiation Act of 1973, and The Education for All Handicapped Children Act of 1975).

The Education for All Handicapped Children Act of 1975 provides funds for several education programs for developmentally disabled and mentally retarded children, but education programs for mentally ill children are not included. The Vocational Rehabilitiation Act of 1973 is specifically directed toward the mentally retarded and toward the physically disabled. Such legislation is responsible for the development of a greater number of community vocational rehabilitiation programs for the mentally retarded than for the mentally ill. A more thorough review of vocational rehabilitation programs indicated that programs were specifically directed toward the mentally retarded. This fact was obvious in the organizational structure of vocational rehabilitation facilities and the type of work available.

Mental health system personnel were also concerned about the lack of psychosocial rehabilitation services for the mentally ill. Most mentally retarded clients had access to training programs for developing daily living skills, managing their homes and finances, using transportation, and socializing. Mentally ill clients did not have the same opportunities.

Differences in federal legislation and eligibility (attributed to several facts) ultimately affected the deinstitutionalization effort. One fact contributing to these differences was the categorical nature of agencies, programs, and services that existed to serve the mental health and mental retardation systems. Another possible fact was that the needs and range of services for the developmentally disabled were better known and easier to define than those for the mentally ill. Furthermore, the lack of data concerning the chronic mentally ill population may have also affected the development and support of federally initiated programs.

Differences in Income Maintenance

Another barrier for the deinstitutionalization process has been the problem in obtaining SSI. Under the current SSI system it is more difficult for the mentally ill to gain assistance in determining disability eligibility than for the mentally retarded to do so. As indicated earlier, the procedures involved in establishing eligibility are frequently lengthy, troublesome, and complex.

One solution to the problem, especially for the mentally ill, is to develop a presumptive eligibility criterion so that payments will not delay community-based placement. Although a person with a developmental disability can readily qualify for presumptive eligibility, a mentally ill individual cannot qualify. This fact has hindered the deinstitutionalization of the mentally ill.

Conclusion

In general, factors that affected the deinstitutionalization process were relevant for both the mental health and mental retardation system. However, the degree and magnitude of problems and barriers for each system varied between states. In spite of the development of community mental health centers and the availability of funds through the Community Support Programs, there are still many changes needed for deinstitutionalizing the mentally ill population.

In order for the deinstitutionalization process to work effectively for the mentally ill, policy and legislative changes must be formulated at the federal level. The financing of community services at the state level should be changed; and, finally, the quantity and quality of programs at the community level should be improved.

6
Recommendations

Suggested Policy Changes
Within the Current System

For more than two years, federal and state agencies and special task forces have identified barriers to the success of deinstitutionalization. Reports issued by General Accounting Office, the Task Force on Deinstitutionalization, and several states, as well as journal articles, provided recommendations for improving the deinstitutionalization process. While many of these recommendations are worthy of support, the time has come to take some action at the national and state levels. Priority issues must be identified; policy and program changes must be implemented; and, finally, a commitment must be made at the federal, state, and local levels to support and enforce the goals and objectives of deinstitutionalization.

A review of journal articles, policy analyses, reports, and state plans concerning the mentally disabled suggests that the problems with, and barriers to, deinstitutionalization have been overidentified. The problems appear to be so numerous, and the difficulties so insurmountable, that little has been done in the way of policy change. Consequently, we have addressed only the issues that we consider to be most vital to the deinstitutionalization effort. The majority of our recommendations for program and policy changes were developed so that they could be implemented and monitored at the federal level.

The following recommendations take into consideration the extremely complex nature of the system. They are offered as a first step toward alleviating specific problems and improving system operation. The recommendations for policy changes within the care-giving system that deals with other than mental health problems were based upon the suggestions of mental health professionals, who may not have always completely understood other elements of the care-giving system.

Administrative or System Issues

As mentioned previously, 60 percent of the respondents identified administrative, managerial, or policy barriers to the achievement of objectives of deinstitutionalization. They reported difficulty in supporting the deinstitutionalization process because on the one hand, service providers are discouraged from institutionalizing the mentally disabled, while on the other hand, very few federal programs are designed to aid the mentally disabled in the community. For instance, the mentally disabled seldom have access to Title XX funds. Furthermore, it is unlikely that this trend will change unless policies and programs at the federal level are changed. In addition, Medicare and Medicaid policies act as disincentives to deinstitutionalization. Finally, the deinstitutionalization effort has been greatly hindered by inconsistencies in federal programs and by the fragmented development of policies at federal and state levels.

The creation of an interdepartmental task force similar to the Deinstitutionalization Task Force seems appropriate. The purpose of this group would be: (1) to identify specific program inconsistencies in legislation, (2) to develop specific changes for *priority* issues, (3) to establish new national deinstitutionalization goals and objectives that would coordinate federal programs and policies, and (4) to provide guidelines for changing legislation. Priority issues for the task force would include: (1) changes in programs and policies for Title XVIII and Title XIX, (2) changes in distributing Title XX social service funds to the mentally disabled, (3) changes in SSI, (4) changes in the development and maintenance of residential facilities (changes in HUD policies), and (5) changes in specific community programs (vocational rehabilitation, special education, and community mental health center programs for the chronically mentally disabled).

In order to further the development of case management services, the task force should examine case management models for use as part of the community support system for chronically disabled individuals. The development of case management services could be encouraged by: (1) providing special long-term funding for such services, (2) providing special training programs in the case management concept, and (3) emphasizing the monitoring of client goal achievement.

Training programs that provide care-giving staffs with the skills necessary to meet the special needs of multidiagnosis clients should be developed and instituted. Incentives to encourage staff members to acquire these skills should also be provided, and clear responsibility for these clients should be assigned.

The national deinstitutionalization goals and objectives should be monitored and evaluated periodically through the office of the Secretary of DHEW, which would review the planning, coordination, and policy implementation of state objectives.

Because Title XX gives states such broad discretion concerning the use of funds, services for deinstitutionalized clients are often created and paid for after most other services. Consideration should be given to expanding Title XX ceilings and requiring states to serve deinstitutionalized clients.

In spite of the vocational rehabilitation mandate to the states to serve the "severely disabled," there still appeared to be problems in getting vocational rehabilitation agencies to serve mentally disabled clients. Priority should be given to vocational programs specifically geared to the needs of these clients and/or the meaning of "severely disabled" should be clarified.

The cost of providing generic services should be considered and calculated in setting up and running any community placement program. At the federal level, provisions should be made for giving funds directly to the states for coordinating, identifying, and filling the gaps in the service delivery system. Although many state plans address this issue, few states have yet received funds for such endeavors. It is possible to use formula grants to support state efforts by adding a section to P.L. 94-63, Section 314(d). Such a provision would help fund the coordination, development, and implementation of the deinstitutionalization plan required under Title I.

Provisions should be made for a state coordinating council (similar to state developmental disabilities councils), which would include representatives from both the mental health and developmental disabilities systems and would be a direct link to federal programs. In addition, the council would establish a state policy (in accordance with national policy) for implementing deinstitutionalization efforts.

Provisions should also be made through the NIMH Community Support Program (CSP) for coordinating, planning, and filling service gaps for the *chronically* mentally disabled. CSP appropriations could be used to start services at the state level. Later, the new services would be maintained through supplements to social service funds under Title XX funding (provided that Title XX increases its funding).

Economic or Cost-Related Issues

Problems with program funding patterns were discussed by 75 percent of the respondents. Although several individuals felt that the amount of funding available was adequate, many thought the program policies and funding mechanisms needed to be directed more toward encouraging community living for the mentally disabled. Specifically, programs such as Medicaid, Medicare, Title XX, and SSI should be changed to make possible the development of more community-based services. For a number of reasons, Title XX funds were rarely used for the mentally disabled. Furthermore, for the mentally ill, Medicare and Medicaid programs encouraged the maintenance of institutions rather than the development of community facilities. Finally, SSI policies have had a negative effect on clients who need access to a wide range of community services and facilities.

The development of funding patterns related to specific client needs appears to be necessary. Existing funding streams, such as those derived from Medicare and Medicaid, created disincentives to deinstitutionalization. Funding support should be decoupled from specific programs, procedures, or target groups and related directly to client needs. Thus, a funding stream specifically designed to support the objectives of deinstitutionalization should be created. As an alternative to the creation of a new program, Title XX ceilings and mandates could be revised so the act could serve as a new funding mechanism.

Program policies and regulations that provide disincentives to deinstitutionalization should be altered. Particularly for the mentally ill, Medicare and Medicaid policies tended to support institutional facilities rather than to encourage the development of community-based services and programs. It appeared that states used Title XVIII and Title XIX funds to upgrade and maintain institutional construction and staffing programs rather than planning reductions in institutional populations and creating community services. On the other hand, if federal funds were limited to institutional type care, patients would be released to inadequate and nonexistent programs in the community. Consequently, the deinstitutionalization movement is at a crossroads: neither the institution nor the community is capable of assuming responsibility for the mentally disabled. However, with changes in the Medicare and Medicaid programs, certain incentives could be created to encourage development of community programs and facilities. The following changes are suggested.

1. Encourage states to utilize Medicare funds for the development and certification of small community facilities.
2. Increase Medicare coverage for noninstitutional treatment for the mentally disabled. Revise the criteria for eligibility to reflect "least restrictive conditions." Medicare coverage should include payment for psychiatric services in the community.
3. Initiate program incentives for institutions to provide outpatient psychiatric care and services, home health care benefits, and psychiatric follow-up and evaluation services to deinstitutionalized Medicare beneficiaries. These activities, when possible, should be coordinated with CMHCs.
4. Remove obstacles and disincentives to the use of Medicare funds by CMHCs and psychiatric clinics.
5. Use Medicaid funds for developing and maintaining small-scale community facilities – for twenty or fewer residents.
6. Evaluate and monitor the use of Medicaid funds for institutional care after they have gone to the states. Determine how these funds could be used to support deinstitutionalization efforts.
7. Provide Medicaid program incentives that would discourage further development and remodeling of institutions and encourage the use of funds for developing community alternatives.
8. Eliminate the unnecessary and inappropriate safety codes (in Title XIX) for small-scale residential facilities.

The revision and simplification of SSI policies and procedures would have a more immediate and direct impact on clients than any changes in other programs. The following should be considered.

1. Complex SSI eligibility requirements should be clarified and/or provisions should be made for presumptive eligibility and automatic eligibility for persons who were eligible for benefits prior to hospitalization.
2. The thirty-day limit on activating SSI eligibility should be extended to maximize the time period in which clients may be placed in the most appropriate community residences.
3. Regulations that require institutionalized clients to lose their SSI eligibility and in effect to lose community residences should be modified; or a provision should be made for a rehabilitative service agency to hold the lease for clients' apartments or residences during this period.
4. Revolving state accounts should be created to support the immediate community placement of persons awaiting determination of their eligibility for SSI.
5. Policies concerning presumptive eligibility should be revised such that those who were eligible for SSI benefits prior to hospitalization maintain their eligibility at discharge.
6. SSI benefits should be continued for individuals receiving temporary (up to three months) hospitalization. The funds would be used to continue payments for community living facilities.
7. Monitoring and evaluation of funds at local agencies should be increased to ensure that recipients are receiving full benefits so that persons receiving SSI grants are aware that they can work and earn more than the maximum without reduction of SSI payments if their work is related to the achievement of self-support.
8. SSA should revise its current definition of mental deficiency to include a specific criterion for measuring adaptive behavior. This criterion would be used for purposes of determining SSI and Social Security eligibility.

9. SSA should improve its relationships and channels of communication with regional, state, and local agencies (that is, improve procedures for informing claimants of the specific reasons for denial of benefits).

Frequently, respondents stated that funding patterns were more closely linked to a kind or range of service than to the needs of clients. Consequently, clients received whatever services could be funded rather than services that were most appropriate. Again, due to the lack of coordination, the confusion regarding program funding, and numerous regulations, the mentally disabled have traditionally been excluded from using Title XX social services because states generally assumed that they received funding from other programs. Although the mentally disabled needed generic services provided by Title XX, they seldom had access to them. As a result, some services were duplicated and other *needed* services were not available. While this situation might have varied from state to state, states generally did not include the mentally disabled in their state plan, or they used their funds for more traditional services (excluding the mentally disabled), or they failed to recognize the national priority of deinstitutionalization efforts. Title XX funds should be used to provide services in support of deinstitutionalization.

An increase in the Title XX budget could promote the development of services for the deinstitutionalization of the chronically mentally disabled. Funds should be provided to residents in sheltered employment, alternative housing arrangements, and day care programs. Finally, Title XX funds should be utilized to provide support services for deinstitutionalized persons.

Social, Legal, and Training Issues

Problems in maintaining and supporting community-based services and facilities were mentioned by 78 percent of the respondents. In addition to citing the fragmentation and gaps in community services, respondents stated that federal legislation, policies, and programs were not designed to accommodate the mentally disabled living in the community. The following changes would improve the provision and operation of community-based services.

1. Categorical funding that discourages the development of some alternatives should be identified and modified since the fullest range of flexible community alternatives should effectively service the needs of clients.
2. HUD application processes that discourage the development of small, normalized community settings should be redesigned.
3. The role played by HUD in providing funds for community alternatives should be increased by: (a) simplifying HUD procedures, (b) providing additional resources to states to better cope with HUD's complexities, or (c) shifting an appropriate proportion of HUD resources to mental health and developmental disabilities budgets.
4. Policies and guidelines for monitoring and evaluating community residential facilities should be examined for areas in which they are either too inflexible to allow clients to live in normalized settings or so loose that quality is lacking.
5. The constitutional right of the mentally disabled to live in any neighborhood should be clearly established by federal policy and reinforced by federal funding policies. For example, evidence of nondiscrimination against the handicapped could be a criterion for dispensing federal funds to localities.
6. The positive impact and costs of involuntary treatment acts should be examined and revisions should be made where appropriate.

Presently, the Community Mental Health Center Program (enacted in 1963) and the Community Mental Health Center Act Amendments of 1975 require the CMHCs to provide basic services—inpatient, outpatient, and emergency care; partial hospitalization; consultation and education; screening; transitional halfway-house services; and follow-up care for residents who have been discharged from a mental health facility in their area. Although these services are required, we do not know the degree to which they are being provided. In addition, the Community Support Program was initiated with the *intent* of increasing services for the chronically mentally disabled. However, it has not been determined if community services have improved for the severely disabled since baseline data on this population is scarce and very little information has been gathered on the service needs of this group.

Multidiagnosis clients are also neglected. In part, because of the development of programs by category, neither developmental disability nor mental health programs take the initiative in providing and maintaining community services for the multiproblem client. The following recommendations should be considered:

1. Review CMHC and Community Support Program applications and monitoring devices to assure that adequate attention is paid to the care of the chronically mentally disabled. Collect data on the size of this population and evaluate the extent to which services are being provided in the CMHC areas.

2. Require all DHEW-funded community mental health centers to provide services to mentally retarded persons with mental and emotional difficulties.

3. Earmark funds to evaluate the collection of data on mental disabilities and to evaluate current programs that link institutional programs to community-based services. Provide funds to agencies to pursue these activities.

4. Develop pilot projects to provide financing for an expanded array of *community treatment* services under Medicare and Medicaid. The projects should be de-

signed to eliminate incentives for unnecessary care in hospitals or nursing homes. Include funds for evaluating and monitoring the project.

5. Provide block grants through legislative changes, to states for mental health services with emphasis on community-based care as recommended by the Deinstitutionalization Task Force.

Due to a lack of community living facilities, the chronically mentally disabled population was still either confined to institutional facilities or forced to live in inadequate, poverty-level residential areas. Although there had been a large increase in the number of community living facilities, the severely disabled continued to have problems obtaining adequate living arrangements. Few managers of board and care and halfway houses wanted to deal with the severely disabled. To improve and increase the number of community residential facilities, federal, state, and local efforts should be intensified to improve the quality of housing and to encourage the development of normalized living facilities. The following recommendations are suggested.

1. Earmark funds for experimental community programs using innovative approaches to serve the mentally disabled. Link these experiments and/or demonstrations to HUD Section 8 "independent group residences." (Section 8: Housing Assistance Payments: Housing and Community Development Act [P.L. 93-383])

2. Review possibilities for providing grants and/or loans from the Small Business Administration of the Economic Development Administration (U.S. Department of Commerce) to capitalize residential situations such as group homes, alternative housing, and sheltered housing facilities on behalf of individuals and groups in the community wishing to participate in such ventures.

3. Budget and provide funds, through the Medicaid program, under appropriate legal and regulatory requirements, to assure that community health-related
facilities are upgraded to meet reasonable community
care standards.

During the site visits, respondents stated that Life Safety
codes required by Title XIX (Medicaid) Intermediate Care
Facility – Mentally Retarded (ICF-MR) regulations were inappropriate and unnecessary for many community residential
facilities. The safety codes, which were originally developed
for institutions, merely encourage the development of mini-
institutions. Enforcement of the safety codes results in higher
construction and maintenance costs, delays in developing
needed facilities, and less desirable (for example, less "normal") living arrangements for the mentally disabled. It is suggested that DHEW establish a departmental task force and
perhaps an advisory committee representing various organizations (for example, the Mental Health Association, National
Association for Retarded Citizens, and National Fire Protection Association) to review inappropriate regulations and suggest changes in the Title XIX Life Safety codes.

Seventy-four percent of the respondents agreed that there
were problems in the delivery of generic services to the mentally disabled and that these problems influenced the operation
of the deinstitutionalization process. There are many reasons
for this situation, including the categorical development of programs (which encourages fragmentation and lack of interagency
cooperation) and the development of programs that are
centered around the type of resources (funding, staffing)
available rather than around the needs of the clients.

The vocational rehabilitation system does not respond to
the needs of deinstitutionalized clients. The following changes
are suggested.

1. Provide special project funds under the Vocational
Rehabilitation Act of 1973 for initiating and developing

"psychosocial rehabilitation services" to be developed through joint planning by state vocational rehabilitation and mental health agencies.

2. Coordinate more closely the goals and objectives of federally funded rehabilitation programs for the mentally disabled under the Vocational Rehabilitation Act of 1973 and Social Security Disability Insurance (SSDI) and SSDI beneficiary rehabilitation programs in order to give an increased number of severely disabled persons access to needed services.

3. Strengthen the role of state vocational rehabilitation agencies in the rehabilitation of SSI recipients by authorizing the use of Title II and Title XVI funds for rehabilitation services leading to increased earnings and an eventual reduction of benefits.

4. Shift vocational rehabilitation and Department of Labor staff support and responsibilities to training needs of the severely mentally disabled.

5. Provide a "success" weighting system for more severely handicapped persons that would reward performance beyond that which is ordinarily expected for each class of disability, so that rehabilitation counselors would be encouraged to provide services for all levels of retarded individuals, including the severely disabled.

6. Earmark CETA Title III funds under discretionary control of the secretary of the Department of Labor for slots for mentally disabled and for support of persons who will work in HUD Section 8 "independent group residences" as resident assistants.

7. Change the U.S. Employment Service (USES) formula to give higher priority to serving the mentally disabled through job counseling and placement services in local USES offices.

8. Remove time limits on CETA slots for either the mentally disabled or persons serving them in "independent group residences."

When discussing educational services for the mentally disabled, 20 percent of the respondents indicated that there were problems with local school districts and federal education programs, particularly for the adult mentally retarded. Recommendations for improving the educational system include:

1. Extend vocational education to adult mentally retarded persons, both in institutions and the community; and monitor enforcement of the rule for assuring that 10 percent of federal education funds apply to the training of handicapped persons.
2. Earmark adult education funds to provide educational and recreational opportunities to mentally disabled persons in such residential situations as nursing homes, halfway houses, independent living centers, and HUD-assisted housing.

In many instances, community-based services were too understaffed to develop and provide services. Furthermore, board and care administrators and facility operators did not feel they were adequately trained, particularly for dealing with the chronically mentally disabled. The following changes are recommended:

1. Allocate funds for the retraining and relocation of institutional staff members and for the relocation of professional staff members to rural areas. Where benefits accrued by employees are not transferable, special funds should be created to compensate for losses.
2. Provide special training programs, both in management and direct service provision, to community services staff. Special attention and incentives should be directed toward helping care-givers to better understand the mentally disabled and meet the special needs of chronic patients. In order to avoid rapid turnover

and to enhance the utility of training programs, special consideration should be given to providing meaningful work and wage incentives for nursing and boarding home staffs.

3. Develop incentives and rewards to encourage operators of board and care facilities and nursing homes to take more difficult clients (for example chronic, acting-out clients) who otherwise may return to institutions.

4. Orient mental health personnel to the kinds of services needed by persons in "independent group residences," and assist state mental health authorities in training resident assistants for service in HUD Section 8 housing arrangements for the mentally disabled.

5. Earmark funds under the service and planning authorities – such as Title XX, Health Resources Administration (HRA), Manpower, CHMCs, Vocational Rehabilitation, Administration on Aging (AOA) – to initiate courses and programs for training personnel who can effect the shift of clients from institutional care to community-based alternatives. These funds should be used not only to retrain current personnel, but also to instruct new personnel. Special emphasis should be placed on retraining those who will lose institutional care jobs as a consequence of the shift from institutional care to the community.

6. Utilize Title XX funds (above the ceiling) for retraining hospital and institutional employees for employment in the community.

System Changes to Improve the
Deinstitutionalization Process

Although most of our recommendations relate to improving the basic operation of the current system, useful prototypes for altering the system were also discovered in the course of this project. It is recommended that potential and operating dynamics of these prototypes be carefully studied to determine what proportion of the chronically disabled population might be served in the future.

Many community placements – nursing homes, board and care facilities, or foster family care arrangements – were said by respondents to share many of the characteristics of institutions. Those facilities tended to reinforce the dependency of clients by caring for many of their needs. The operators of these facilities received many incentives to maintain dependency rather than "graduating" clients to higher levels of self-sufficiency. That is, much "community placement" for the chronically disabled appears to be "mini-institutional placement." The danger is that clients will continue to develop dependency and, over the long term, their ability to function self-sufficiently will deteriorate.

One alternative to traditional, often mini-institutional placements is psychosocial rehabilitation programs, which have existed for many years but are not numerous, mainly because policies that determine reimbursement have kept them out of the main funding streams for deinstitutionalized clients. Rather than taking the "normal" environment as a given and expending effort to fit the disabled individual into it, these programs create small, viable social systems that better meet the total life needs of individuals whose capabilities and needs constitute a long-term deviation from the conventional norm. These programs attempt to create an environment in which chronically disabled individuals can maximize their potentials for self-determination, self-care, productivity, and the enjoyment of life. In addition to encouraging maximum feasible self-sufficiency for clients, psychosocial programs also emphasize the clients' contribution toward the operation of the support system. The latter consideration is extremely important for keeping the costs of an extensive support system within reasonable bounds.

Psychosocial rehabilitation models should be examined in light of the following questions.

1. What models for nondependency-inducing support systems are currently in operation?
2. In what ways could the usage of those models be expanded?
3. By what process are clients placed in community support systems?
4. How many and what kinds of chronically disabled clients need continuing support services?
5. What proportion of these clients could be served by the existing models?
6. What proportion of these clients could be served by models that could be made available?
7. What are the relative costs of conventional community placements and the models?
8. What policies related to funding, facility standards, housing, or staffing standards would need to be altered in order to make operation of the models feasible?

These are complex questions that cannot be fully answered given our present knowledge. However, attempts must be made to answer these questions and to develop a conceptual framework within which further empirical investigations can be carried out.

References

Amicus. 1977. National Center for Law and the Handicapped. 2, 6 (November): South Bend, Ind.

Arnoff, F. N. 1975. "Social consequences of policy toward mental illness." *Science* 188:1277-1281.

Aviram, U., and Segal, S. P. 1973. "Exclusion of the mentally ill: reflection on an old problem in a new context." *Archives of General Psychiatry* 29:126-131.

Bachrach, L. L. 1976. *Deinstitutionalization: an analytic review and sociological perspective.* Washington, D.C.: U.S. Government Printing Office.

———. 1976a. "A note on some recent studies of released mental hospital patients in the community." *American Journal of Psychiatry* 133:73-75.

Barnett, C. R. 1975. "An anthropologist's perspective." In *Humanizing health care,* eds. J. Howard and A. Strauss. New York: John Wiley & Sons.

Barton, R. 1966. *Institutional neurosis.* 2d ed. Bristol: John Wright & Sons.

Bassuk, E. L., and Gerson, S. 1978. "Deinstitutionalization and mental health services." *Scientific American* 238:46-53.

Becker, A., and Schulberg, C. 1976. "Phasing out state hospitals — psychiatric dilemma." *New England Journal of Medicine* 294: 255-261.

Binner, P. R. 1977. "Deinstitutionalization: an analysis of the problem." Unpublished manuscript. Denver: University of Denver, Denver Research Institute.

Bonn, E. M.; Binner, P. R.; and Huber, H. M. 1975. "Evaluation of a modern state hospital: the Fort Logan Mental Health Center experience." In *The future role of the state hospital,* eds. J. Zusman and E. F. Bertsch. Lexington, Mass: D. C. Heath & Co.

Borus, J., et al. 1975. "The coordination of mental health services at the neighborhood level." *The American Journal of Psychiatry* 132, 11:1177–1181.

Bruininks, R. H.; Thurlow, M. L.; Williams, S. M.; and Morveau, L. E. 1978. *Deinstitutionalization and residential services: a literature review.* Project report no. 1. Minneapolis: University of Minnesota.

California Department of Health. 1974. *Report and recommendations on the impact of local zoning ordinances on community care facilities.* Sacramento, Calif.

————. 1978. *Old problems, new directions.* Report of the 1978/79 Budget Augmentation for Mental Health. Sacramento, Calif.

Chodoff, P. 1976. "The case for involuntary hospitalization of the mentally ill." *American Journal of Psychiatry* 133:496–501.

Chu, F. D., and Trotter, S. 1972. *The mental health complex. Part I: community mental health centers.* Washington, D.C.: Center for Study of Responsive Law.

Conroy, J. W. 1977. "Trends in deinstitutionalization." *Mental Retardation* 15, 4:44–46.

Curtis, R. W., and Herskowitz, J. 1977. *Deinstitutionalization and its effect on employees.* Taunton, Mass.: Social Matrix Research.

Datel, W. E., and Murphy, J. G. 1976. "A cost-benefit analysis of community versus institutional living." *Hospital and Community Psychiatry* 27, 3:165–170.

Datel, W. E.; Murphy, J. G.; and Pollack, P. L. 1978. "Outcome in a deinstitutionalization program employing service integration methodology." *Journal of Operational Psychiatry* 9, 1:6–24.

Demone, W., and Schulberg, C. 1975. "Has the state mental hospital a future as a human service resource?" In *The future role of the state hospital,* eds. J. Zusman and E. F. Bertsch. Lexington, Mass.: D. C. Heath & Co.

Deutsch, A. 1948. *Shame of the states.* New York: Harcourt, Brace & Co.

Dingman, P. R. 1974. "The case for the state mental hospital." In *Where is my home?* Proceedings of a Conference on the Closing of State Mental Hospitals, ed. Stanford Research Institute. Menlo Park, Calif. Stanford Research Institute.

Etzioni, A. 1975. "Deinstitutionalization. A public policy fashion." *Human Behavior* 4 (September):12–13.

Flaschner, F. N. 1975. "Constitutional requirements in commitment of the mentally ill: rights to liberty and therapy." In *The future role of the state hospital,* eds. J. Zusman and E. F. Bertsch. Lexington, Mass. : D. C. Heath & Co.

Glenn, T. D. 1975. "Community programs for chronic patients – administrative financing." *Psychiatric Annals* 5:175.

Goffman, E. 1961. *Asylums.* New York: Doubleday.

Greenblatt, M. 1957. "Implications for psychiatry and hospital practice: the movement from custodial hospital to therapeutic community." In *The patient and the mental hospital,* eds. M. Greenblatt, D. J. Levinson, and R. H. Williams. Glencoe, Ill. Free Press.

Greenblatt, M., and Glazier, E. 1975. "The phasing out of mental hospitals in the United States." *American Journal of Psychiatry* 132:1135–1140.

Group for the Advancement of Psychiatry, Committee on Psychiatry and the Community. 1978. *The Chronic Mental Patient in the Community.* New York: Mental Health Materials Center, Inc.

Gruenberg, E. M. 1967. "The social breakdown syndrome – some origins." *American Journal of Psychiatry* 123:1481–1489.

Gunderson, J. 1974. "Special report: schizophrenia, 1974." *Schizophrenia Bulletin* (Summer):16–54.

Hailey, A. M. 1971. "Long-stay psychiatric inpatients: a study based on the Camberwell Register." *Psychological Medicine* 1:128.

Halpert, H. P. 1969. "Public acceptance of the mentally ill." *Public Health Reports* 84:59–64.

Herbert, W. 1977. "Seeking the missing rungs." *APA Monitor* 8, 7:1–11.

Horizon House Institute for Research and Development. 1975. "The future role of state mental hospitals: a national survey of planning and program trends." Philadelphia.

Illinios Commission on Mental Health and Developmental Disabilities. 1976. "Mental health '77, a system in transition: annual report 1976–77." Springfield, Ill.

Joint Commission on Mental Illness and Health. 1961. *Action for Mental Health.* New York: Basic Books.

Karls, J. 1976. "Retraining hospital staff for work in community programs in California." *Hospital and Community Psychiatry* 27: 262–265.

Kennedy, J. F. 1963. "President John F. Kennedy's Special Message to the Congress on Mental Health and Mental Retardation." Washington, D. C.: U.S. Government Printing Office, February 5, 1963.

Kirk, S. A., and Therrien, M. E. 1975. "Community mental health myths and the fate of former hospitalized patient." *Psychiatry* 38 (August):209–217.

Klerman, G. L. 1977. "Better but not well: social and ethical issues in the deinstitutionalization of the mentally ill." *Schizophrenia Bulletin* 3, 4:617–631.

Koenig, P. 1978. "Problem that can't be tranquilized." *New York Times Magazine,* May 21, 1978.

Kramer, M. 1977. "Psychiatric services and the changing institutional scene, 1950–1985." DHEW Publication No. (ADM) 77-433, Series 13, No. 12. Washington, D.C.: Department of Health, Education, and Welfare, National Institute of Mental Health.

Lamb, H. R., and Goertzel, V. 1971. "Discharged mental patients— are they really in the community?" *Archives of General Psychiatry* 24:29–34.

McGuire, P. A. 1978. "Fort Logan: turning into a human warehouse." *Denver Post,* April 2, 1978, "Contemporary," pp. 6–10.

McPartland, S., and Richard, H. 1966. "Analysis of readmissions to a community mental health center." *Community Mental Health Journal 2,* 1:22–26.

Markson, E. W. 1976. "Massachusetts: comparisons and contrasts, a review of deinstitutionalization outcomes." Prepared for presentation at the American Orthopsychiatric Association, Atlanta, Ga., March 5, 1976.

Markson, E. W., and Cumming, J. H. 1976. "The post-transfer fate of relocated patients." In *State mental hospitals,* eds. P. I. Ahmed and S. C. Plog. New York: Plenum Publishing Co.

Marlowe, R. A. 1972. "Effects of relocating geriatric state hospital patients." Paper presented at the 25th Annual Meeting of the Gerontology Society, San Juan, Puerto Rico, December 1972.

Mendel, W. M. 1974. "Dismantling the mental hospital." In *Where is my home?* Proceedings of a Conference on the Closing of State Mental Hospitals, ed. Stanford Research Institute. Menlo Park, Calif.: Stanford Research Institute.

Moser, L. R.; Menn, A.; and Matthews, S. M. 1975. "Soteria: evaluation of a home based treatment for schizophrenia." *American Journal of Orthopsychiatry* 45:455–467.

National Center for Health Statistics. 1977. *Nursing Homes in the United States: 1973–1974, National Nursing Home Survey.* Washington, D.C.: U.S. Department of Health, Education, and Welfare.

National Institute of Mental Health. 1976. "Community living arrangements for the mentally disabled: issues and options for public policy." Proceedings of a Working Conference. Washington, D.C.: U.S. Department of Health, Education, and Welfare, Alcohol, Drug Abuse, and Mental Health Administration.

Ozarin, L. 1976. "Community alternatives to institutional care." *American Journal of Psychiatry* 133:69–72.

Pattakos, A. 1976. "Efficacy of mental health employees in an era of deinstitutionalization of state hospitals." *Journal of Collective Negotiations* 5, 3:225–232.

Polak, P. R., and Kirby, M. 1976. "A model to replace psychiatric hospitals." *Journal of Neurosis and Mental Disease* 162:13–22.

Polak, P. R.; Deeber, S.; and Kirby, M. 1977. "On treating the insane in sane places." *Journal of Community Psychology* 5:380–387.

President's Committee on Mental Retardation. 1976. *MR '76: Mental retardation past and present.* Washington, D.C.: U.S. Government Printing Office.

Rabkin, J. 1974. "Public attitudes toward mental illness: a review of the literature." *Schizophrenia Bulletin* 10 (Fall):9–33.

Reding, G. R. 1974. Letter in *Psychiatric News*, May 1, 1974.

Rieder, R. O. 1974. "Hospitals, patients, and politics." *Schizophrenia Bulletin* 11 (Winter):9–14.

Sanders, D. H. 1972. "Innovative environments in the community: a life for the chronic patient." *Schizophrenia Bulletin* 6 (Fall): 49–59.

Scheerenberger, R. C. 1974. "A model for deinstitutionalization." *Mental Retardation* 12, 6:3–7.

Slovenko, R., and Luby, E. D. 1974. "From moral treatment to railroading out of the mental hospital." *Bulletin of the American Academy of Psychiatry and the Law* 2 (December):223–236.

Smith, B. J. 1974. "A hospital support system for chronic patients living in the community." *Hospital and Community Psychiatry* 25:508–509.

Soskin, R. M. 1977. "The least restrictive alternative: in principle and in application." *Amicus* 2, 6:28–32.

Stanton, A. H., and Schwartz, M. S. 1954. *The mental hospital: a study of institutional participation in psychiatric illness and treatment.* New York: Basic Books.

State of Florida, Department of Health and Rehabilitative Services, Mental Health Program Office. 1978. "Deinstitutionalization concept paper." Tallahassee, Fla.

Stein, L. and Test, M. A. 1976. "Retraining hospital staff for work in a community program in Wisconsin." *Hospital and Community Psychiatry* 27:266–268.

Steinhart, M. J. 1973. "The selling of community mental health." *Psychiatric Quarterly* 47:325–340.

Trotter, S., and Kuttner, B. 1974. "The mentally ill: from back wards to back alleys." *Washington Post,* February 24, 1974.

U.S., Congress, House. 1976. *Hearing* before the House Subcommittee on Health and Long-Term Care of the Select Committee on Aging, 94th Cong., 2d sess., September 30, 1976.

U.S., Department of Health, Education, and Welfare, National Institute of Mental Health, Division of Biometry. n.d. *Statistical Note #74.* Washington, D. C.

U.S., Department of Health, Education, and Welfare, National Institute of Mental Health, Division of Biometry. 1974. *Statistical Note #110.* Washington, D.C.

U.S., General Accounting Office, Comptroller General of the United States. 1977. *Returning the mentally disabled to the community: government needs to do more.* Washington, D.C.

Wing, J. K. 1962. "Institutionalism in mental hospitals." *British Journal of Social and Clinical Psychology* 1:38–51.

Wolpert, J.; Dear, M.; and Drawford, R. 1974. "Mental health satelite facilities in the community." Presented at the National Institute of Mental Health, Center for Studies of Metropolitan Problems Program Series. Rockville, Md.: U.S. Department of Health, Education, and Welfare, National Institute of Mental Health.

Wyatt v. *Stickney,* 325 F Supp. 781 (M.D. Ala. 1971).

World Health Organization. 1953. *Third report of the Expert Committee on Mental Health.* Technical report series no. 73. Geneva.

Zorber, M. A. 1978. "Residential setting for mentally retarded persons: a review of the literature that assesses policy related residential characteristics and personal adjustment." Unpublished draft paper. Massachusetts Association for Retarded Citizens, n.p.

Zusman, J., and Bertsch, E. F., eds. 1975. *The future role of the state hospital.* Lexington, Mass.: D. C. Heath & Co.

Index